Transformation

Unlock Your True Potential

Dr. Eyad H. Yehyawi

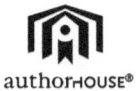

authorHOUSE®

AuthorHouse™
1663 Liberty Drive, Suite 200
Bloomington, IN 47403
www.authorhouse.com
Phone: 1-800-839-8640

First published by AuthorHouse 4/11/2008

ISBN: 978-1-4343-7881-1 (sc)

Printed in the United States of America
Bloomington, Indiana

This book is printed on acid-free paper.

__Transformation__ was written as a sensible guide to help you understand and apply basic physiology, nutrition, training and supplementation to reach your physique goals. Many training principles in this manual are intense, so please have a complete physical and consult with your physician before starting any exercise program or supplement. __Proceed with suggested diets, supplements, and training programs at your own risk.__

Dedicated to my loving parents, who always let me chase my dreams.

"Every person is the creation of themselves, the image of their own thinking and believing."

-Anonymous

Contents

Forward   ix

Introduction   xi

My Story   xi

Let's Get Started   1

Hormones: The Major Players   5

The Macronutrients-
Carbohydrates/Protein/Fats   21

Supplementation   43

Creating the Ideal Nutrition
and Supplement Program   63

Training: The Eight Principles   95

Cardiovascular and Weight Training
to Maximize Fat Loss   135

The Programs   149

Forward

"Desire is the greatest ingredient to being the best there is or ever will be."

-Anonymous

Two years ago, in Cleveland, Ohio, I first entertained the thought of writing this book. My goal was simple. To simplify change, to show people how to manipulate what they ate and how they trained to make significant changes in their bodies. I was fortunate in that while pursuing my dreams of becoming a doctor, I learned a vast amount in regards to nutrition, how the body reacts to stress, and nutrient timing. Still, I never found time to put these thoughts into words.

The years past and I helped many of my friends and clients as a personal trainer. Desire was rarely a problem for those I trained but rather, they didn't quite know where to start. The vast amount of information out there made it difficult to know whose advice to follow and trust. The hundreds of magazines and books all had valuable information, but often, it was overwhelming. Nevertheless, I took it upon myself to read everything that came out in the literature, and while doing so, learned a great deal. It truly was a passion of mine and I wanted to learn as much as I possibly could. At the same time, much of what I read was misleading and yielded poor results. I experimented with countless training and nutrition protocols, either succeeded or failed, but made sure I learned from each experience.

After recovering from an unfortunate medical condition in 2005, I decided that if I was able to workout again, that I would take it to the next level and never look back. Eventually I did start working out again and rebuilding my physique. In the months that followed, I experienced mental and physical changes that I had never encountered before. I was eventually able to share my story with hundreds of individuals through travel, email, and phone. One day while flipping through a magazine, I read a quote by Michael Landon, the famous actor who lost a courageous battle to cancer many years ago. He said, "I wish we would all be told the day we are born that we are dying. That way, we all would live like there was no tomorrow." I decided that day to start working towards completing this book.

The goal was simply to write a book that dismissed all the things I felt didn't work and focus on the things that did. The same techniques I used to reach my goals. *This book is not necessarily a specific program, but rather an understanding of principles that will allow you to reach your ultimate goals.* Too many times we can't perform a program as stated in a magazine or book and feel we won't achieve the results we desire. We all have different schedules, lifts we enjoy, recovery abilities, and physiques we want to attain. Building muscle and losing fat all boils down to the stimulus we place on our body and the nutrients we put into it. As long as you understand these two things, and know them well, you can attain any physique you desire.

Introduction

In late June of 2005, I was finishing my residency at the St. Louis VA hospital when my life changed forever. After helping a student perform an exam, I stood up but could not feel my right leg. I ignored the problem, thinking that my leg had fallen asleep. However, thirty minutes later the feeling had still not returned. I had trouble walking but still was in denial. Fortunately, a fellow doctor talked me into going to the ER where further testing revealed that at the age of 28, I had experienced a stroke.

The following days in the hospital were the four worst days of my life. They did not know what had caused it or what to expect. I tried to stay positive but couldn't help wondering why this had happened to me. I was a two-sport athlete in college, was constantly on the go, and worked out religiously. I had become a personal trainer in 1999 and then pursued my dreams of becoming a doctor. After graduating from optometry school, I pursued advanced training through a pathology residency program for an additional year. So, with one week to go in my residency, and my career just beginning, the unfortunate event took place.

The doctors eventually determined that I had a congenital heart defect. Unfortunately, a small clot that normally would have passed, escaped through this defect, and caused the damage. I soon regained the feeling in my leg but the advice I later received from doctors was crushing. They said that due to the small opening in my heart, any heavy lifting could cause another stroke. I was lucky they told me, but the next time the clot could lodge in another area of my brain, causing permanent damage or death. I had prided myself on staying in shape and had maintained my training, even through the years obtaining my doctorate. Still, I felt as though I had done something wrong, although I had never used steroids or illegal drugs. I was finally released from the hospital with a much different outlook on life.

Two weeks later I finally got the courage to go for a jog and broke down in tears. I was so scared it would happen again. In the weeks that followed I would casually jog or do pushups, but just couldn't bring myself to really "workout." Time passed and I grew more depressed. I could feel my confidence and muscle tone shrinking, while my body fat increased. It was months later when I talked to a doctor that was a close friend of my cousin, also in the medical field. This physician was a neurologist and explained that an incident like this could indeed occur again, but that it had been present since birth, and even with my active lifestyle, I had never experienced any other problems. He told me to return to lifting sensibly and continue treatment with my blood thinner. Before I left he asked me, "Are you really living right now by not doing what you love?"

I immediately went out and bought a journal. *Most importantly I made a promise to myself.* I did not want to compete with anyone else, but rather maximize the potential that my body possessed. I told myself that no matter what the results might be, I would finish what I started and never look back. This was a second chance. Taking the before picture was not a fun experience, but I had to do it. It was a powerful motivator. Looking at it was a reminder of what I had endured and also what I had become. I was well over 16% body fat, overweight, and in poor health, both mentally and physically. Initially, I had trouble running very long and my strength had plummeted. I was determined though. I read everything I could, ate properly, and trained like it was my last day on earth.

In the months that followed I noticed physical and mental changes every day. I paid attention to what I ate, how I trained, and the results soon followed. Just over one year later, I competed in a natural bodybuilding competition and was in better shape than I had ever been. Throughout the entire ordeal I learned a valuable lesson. *No matter the situation, you just can't give up.* In the months following my stroke I had accepted defeat and just went on "living." Please don't ever do that. You can always work around obstacles and be better for it. I wanted to share my story so others can realize it is never too late. I never gave up on my dream of staying fit and neither should you. The incident was a wake up call and made me grateful for everything in my life. I have come to realize that it isn't what happens to us in life that makes us who we are, but how we handle it.

Now, as I write this, _my goal is to help anyone out there who desires to be better_. Maybe it's just to get in better shape for a wedding, a bodybuilding competition, or a reunion. Maybe it's to have a healthier outlook on life for your kids or spouse. Or perhaps, there are just those out there who want to learn more about physiology, training, and nutrition, simply because it interests them. No matter where or who you are, you <u>CAN</u> reach your physique goals and learn something from this manual. After reading this book, you will have a thorough understanding of hormones, nutrition, supplementation, and training. You will also be able to adjust your training and diet to specifically transform your body into what you want. All the tools you need to attain your goals are outlined in this book. It was written for you.

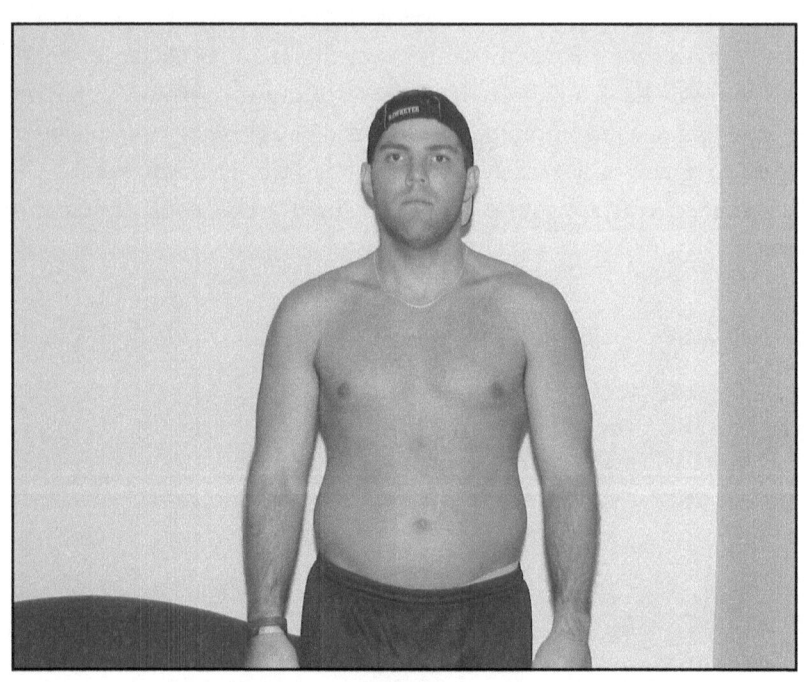

Before

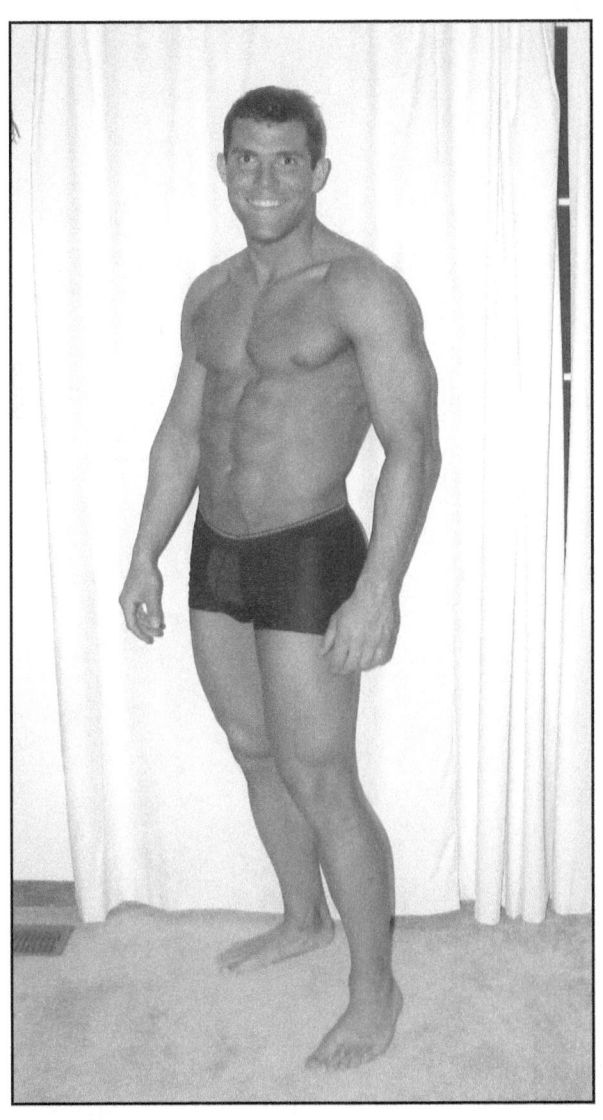

After

Chapter 1

Women and Lifting...Let's get it Straight

I am simply adding this section before the women reading this book think it is written strictly for men. The nutrition, cardio, and training protocols in this manual are written for natural athletes of both sexes. Many women fear getting bigger and masculine looking if they lift weights and that is the furthest thing from the truth. Many of the professional bodybuilding women that are bigger and extremely muscular are not natural and take chemical substances to greatly increase muscle mass. This is the reason the majority of men are naturally more muscular than women-hormone profiles. Unless women use illegal drugs, they will not become extremely muscular and bulky. In actuality, with proper nutrition and training, they will attain a lean and streamlined physique that most all would love to have. Just look at some of the women in fitness. All of them lift and train intensely, I promise! The way to attain this look is with proper nutrition, lifting, and cardiovascular training regimens. This book, regardless of sex, will help you understand nutrition and training, the way the body changes, and how to maximize your natural abilities.

A Basic Understanding

We need to start by understanding a few things related to the physiology of our bodies that have a major impact on how we look. It doesn't matter if our goal is to get leaner and toned, or more muscular and bigger. The fact is the body loves stability. It will do anything and everything to stay where it is and place itself into a safer environment. Fat is protective, and muscle is expensive. Fat provides a source to obtain energy from in times when food is scarce. You see the body doesn't know it's 2007, it has no clue that there is a fast food joint on every corner. So, what does the body think when you eat at 8 am and then not again until 5 pm? That food is scarce and it better prepare for the worse. This, by the way, includes holding onto to as much body fat as it possibly can. The body doesn't know if you finally found something to eat after hunting for hours or if you are just too busy to eat. It only knows how many times you have eaten, and thus eases its mind, or prepares for the worst.

Think of it this way, if you got paid every three hours, would it bother you to spend some cash every day? Now, what if you only got paid every so often, you would be much less inclined to spend money repeatedly and foolishly. The body views fat and food the same way. If you eat every few hours, the body will realize it needs to quickly and efficiently metabolize the food you have eaten as more is coming soon. It also knows it can use this "extra fuel" for tasks that in a state of starvation, may not seem so important, such as building muscle. When we feed our bodies consistently, there is less need to store fat, as a fresh supply of energy will be on its way soon. Essentially our metabolism increases. The opposite of course is true. When you starve the body, it will do everything it can to hold onto as much body fat as possible, as well as store more nutrients as fat! It assumes it won't eat again for many hours and needs a safety reserve. Therefore our metabolism decreases. The bottom line, and one of the first things we must come to terms with is this: **we must eat small meals regularly to increase our metabolism and lose weight.**

Now, in relation to strength training and muscle building, the body is even tougher to trick. We see muscle as something we need in order to look and feel better. The body sees it as a privilege. Muscle is extremely demanding, it requires a great deal of energy to keep it running, and that is why the body sees it as "extra credit". At the same time, adding muscle dramatically increases metabolism and burns fat, even at rest! So if our goal is to lose body fat and gain muscle, we must realize there is only one way to do this. *We must force the body to change through our training programs.* To accomplish this, the training must be intense enough to make the body realize it must adapt, by growing stronger and more efficient. The body must perceive any stimulus as such before it will make significant changes in its structure. If you don't give the body a reason to get bigger, faster, stronger, or lose weight, it just won't! Therefore we must come to terms with another important point: **we must train regularly and intensely to force our bodies to change.**

Ok, so how do we do this? How do we get the body to actually gain muscle and lose fat? We are going to talk about all that in detail in the coming chapters. The key at this time is to realize the two most important points in this book: that **it is vital to eat small meals frequently throughout the day, and that you must have an intense training protocol to force the body to change.** Once we understand that, all we need to do is focus on the training techniques we perform, and the types of nutrients we consume. Consistency in our training and nutrition must follow, and in so doing, your goals will be attained.

Reality Check

Gaining muscle is not that easy. In fact, it's damn hard. Many of you might want to put this book down now and say, "I just want to get in better shape, not put on tons of muscle." Well, if you're worried about gaining "tons" of muscle, and can figure out how to do that quickly, as a natural athlete, you can quit your job and make millions. It's just not that easy. I have been training hard for years and have had to work for every inch of progress. It hasn't been easy but once the changes start, they keep coming! *__Transforming your body is a journey and not a quick fix__*. Once you do get there though, it will be hard to go back as your body will then have a new set point.

To dispel the myth again, muscle gains will do nothing but tone us up and help us lose fat. I promise. Muscle takes energy to keep it running, so the more you have, the less fat you'll accumulate. Even if you put on two pounds of muscle, you will look amazingly better and have a dramatically faster metabolism. Replace the fat with muscle and the scale might be the same but the mirror sure won't! Trust me, even the harshest advocates of not wanting to gain muscle still want to look better, and the techniques in this book can get you there. Those who don't train with weights and simply "starve" themselves are destined to not only put the weight on again one day, but will simply be a smaller version of their previous selves.

I know a lot of athletes who paid the price years ago to gain healthy and appealing amounts of muscle and now only lift occasionally. Surprisingly though, they don't put on much fat as the muscle they possess is so metabolically demanding it prevents fat accumulation. So the bottom line is, male or female, if we want to tone up and lose fat, we must lift weights and gain muscle to get there.

Compete with Yourself

One of the most frustrating parts of some magazines today is the promotion of physiques that were attained with the use of illegal drugs. These include steroids, insulin, human growth hormone (HGH), and testosterone. Not only are these physiques un-natural and un-appealing to many individuals, but the effects these substances have on the body are devastating. This book has no interest in discussing the use of illegal drugs, other than the fact that we must all realize we can attain impressive physiques without these exogenous substances. Although they aid many athletes, we can produce what we need naturally while not putting our health in jeopardy.

So many young bodybuilders, athletes, and the youth of America see these physiques and feel worthless when they can't achieve the same results. That to me is sad. In actuality, these physiques have been penalized of late as bodybuilding is losing its aesthetic qualities. The physiques of the "old days" wouldn't even place by today's standards and that is a shame. **The point here is that we should all focus on us, what we as individuals want, and are capable of.** Lift and eat right, and you will do nothing but improve your health and create a lean, toned physique.

I thought long and hard about what topic should start this book. Everybody wants to talk training and supplements. However, I really feel that to properly discuss those topics, you must understand the body that you are trying to change. If we don't understand how the natural hormones we produce affect our training and nutrition, we will never maximize our physical potential. In saying that, lets start by briefly discussing the major hormones and how they affect our physique.

Chapter 2

HORMONES: THE MAJOR PLAYERS

I included this section first, because it is vital to understand the major hormones in our body and how they affect us. Once you have a solid understanding of these hormones, the training, foods you select, and times you workout, all can be adjusted to yield the greatest results.

Testosterone and Insulin

Many of us think of **testosterone** when we think of hormones that build muscle. Although testosterone is a major component to muscle gains, insulin is just as important. The word **insulin** though often brings visions of diabetes and poor health. What most of us fail to realize however is that although it does aid a large part of the diabetic population, it is also the most anabolic, or muscle building hormone we produce.

The Basics of Testosterone

Let's first discuss testosterone. Testosterone is produced in the testes or ovaries, and is responsible for many of the physical characteristics of males and females. It is found in greater concentrations in men, and that is one reason they naturally produce more muscle. Therefore, it seems to get all the "muscle-building" attention. In fact, women only produce a fraction of the testosterone that men due daily! Without testosterone, we wouldn't have a sex drive, produce muscle, or go through all those fun things like hair loss, acne, and mood swings. It is a necessity, whether we like it or not. An interesting fact related to testosterone is *that it is synthesized from cholesterol*. That's right, the very thing you've always been told to avoid! But I'm here to tell you it's not a bad thing. **The body produces cholesterol daily** and not only is it responsible for natural testosterone production, but it is essential to life. Let's look at the relationship between cholesterol and testosterone a little closer.

The Necessity of Cholesterol and Testosterone

Overall, cholesterol has a bad reputation secondary to its association with heart disease. However, of the two cholesterol variations most commonly discussed, only one should be considered "un-healthy," and that is **low-density lipoprotein (LDL)**. The other, **high-density lipoprotein (HDL)**, often referred to as the "good" cholesterol, is the type we want to make sure we have adequate amounts of. So how do we synthesize cholesterol and where does it come from? Well, we can consume it in its pure form as in egg yolks, but we can also synthesize it after consuming saturated fat. Saturated fat is most commonly found in red meat and cheese, but also is present in egg yolks. Once saturated fat is eaten, it is transported to the liver where it is synthesized into cholesterol.

Then What?

In any case, after cholesterol is either consumed or synthesized in the liver from saturated fat, it then hooks up with its protein carrier and together forms LDL. You see, without a "carrier" it really is useless, and needs a way to travel around the body. That's where LDL and HDL come in, as they are transporters of "bad" and "good" cholesterol. LDL is necessary to "drop" cholesterol off at certain sites so that it can perform vital functions in the body, one of which is the formation of testosterone. Where does HDL come in? Well, its job is to remove the excess cholesterol from the blood stream and transports it back to the liver. That is why we need to ensure it is present in sufficient amounts so that it can clear our blood of excess cholesterol (Fig 1).

Figure 1: Basic Flow Chart of Cholesterol/Testosterone Metabolism

Eat Saturated Fat → Converted to cholesterol in liver → Combines with protein carrier to form LDL → LDL drops cholesterol off at various sites to perform needed functions (ie testosterone production) → HDL clears blood of excess cholesterol and transports it back to the liver where it can be excreted.

Although LDL, cholesterol, and saturated fats are usually deemed unhealthy, we still need them to produce testosterone and perform various other biological functions. **So a _limited amount_ of saturated fat and cholesterol in our diet is actually beneficial!** Healthy levels of HDL ensure that any excess cholesterol is transported out of our blood and back to the liver. It **is those of us who eat saturated fat/cholesterol in excess and do not exercise that problems arise**. In these situations, the amount of LDL's far exceed that which the body needs or can clear out, and it begins to affect our health in a negative way. Although cholesterol and fat are essential to produce adequate amounts of testosterone and support other bodily functions, *they should never be consumed in excess or that which puts our health in jeopardy.*

Important Note:

If you are reading this and have high or uncontrolled LDL, total cholesterol, and/or triglyceride levels, please consult with your physician before thinking that "somebody" told you they are good for you. Your health should be in check before starting any exercise or nutrition protocol and until your blood chemistries are in check, care should be taken in the amount of cholesterol and saturated fat you consume. Once that occurs though, I firmly believe they are a necessity for transforming your physique and ensuring adequate hormone production.

Where Do We Get It

Adequate and *healthy* amounts of cholesterol can be obtained by consuming egg yolks and lean red meats. Again, whole eggs (yolks specifically) contain cholesterol <u>and</u> saturated fat, among other healthy fats, vitamins and minerals. We will discuss these specific fats in more detail later, but for now, realize that healthy amounts of cholesterol and fats are a necessity to build the physique you desire. On the flip side, obesity, over indulgence in saturated fat and cholesterol, and a lack of exercise can severely put your health at risk. Balance and knowledge is the key. Specifically in regards to testosterone, lack of sleep, zero fat intake and over-training all decrease testosterone production. Understanding how cholesterol and fat ensure adequate testosterone production is the first step in understanding the natural production of hormones.

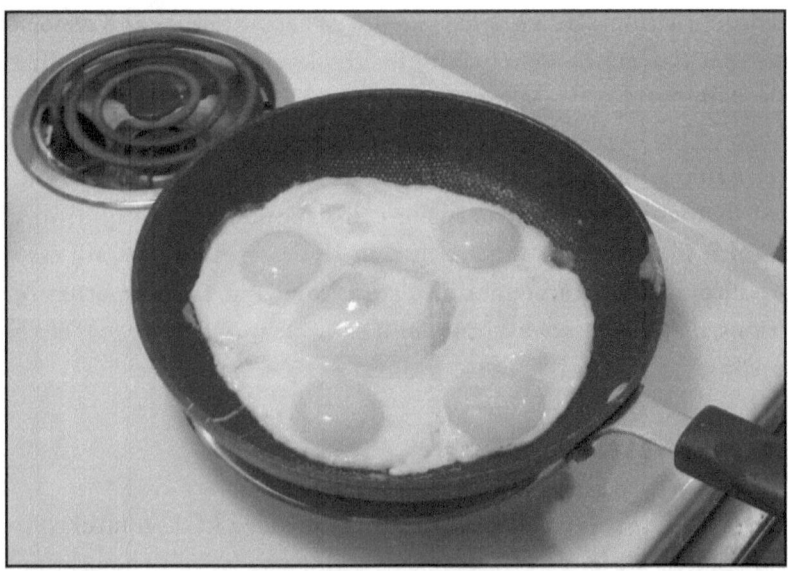

Eggs are a great source of protein and healthy fats. The cholesterol they contain can also aid in natural testosterone production.

The Basics of Insulin

Now, although testosterone is anabolic, or muscle building, we can't control testosterone as well as insulin. In fact, in regards to testosterone, all we can really do is train hard, and consume adequate amounts of red meat and cholesterol to make sure we produce enough natural testosterone. It is however our ability to manipulate insulin that will allow us to maximize fat loss and muscle gains to the greatest extent.

Insulin is produced by the beta cells of the pancreas and allows the nutrients we take in to be used by our body. It can also be our worst enemy, if our goal is to get leaner and decrease body fat. The key is knowing how and when to naturally manipulate the output of this potent hormone. Carbohydrates are the foods most likely to cause an insulin release as they are broken down into our primary energy source called glucose, often referred to as blood sugar. Glucose, as well as fat and protein eventually led to ATP (adenosine triphosphate) production, which is our major energy source. For the purposes of this book, we will simply refer to glucose, fats and proteins as energy sources, knowing that ATP production will soon follow.

Any time we eat, specifically carbohydrates such as breads, cereals, or pasta, we convert them into glucose, and the pancreas releases insulin (see Fig 2). The purpose of insulin then is to shuttle the glucose into the muscles and liver, to eventually be stored as glycogen. **If these stores are filled, the liver will convert excess glucose into fat and transport them to fat cells for storage.**

Fig. 2

Eat "Carbs" → which are broken into glucose → body then releases insulin → which stores glucose as glycogen in the liver and muscles or converts glucose to fat → this leads to ATP production through various processes.

Glycogen and fat are essentially stored energy and can be used for fuel later. How are they used later? Well, another hormone released by the alpha cells of the pancreas, called **glucagon,** is released when blood sugar levels drop and energy is needed. This hormone can initiate fat breakdown, as well as converting glycogen back into glucose. Once this occurs they are dispensed back it into the bloodstream, so we again have a source of energy (see Fig 3). **Simply stated, insulin is released to store energy, and glucagon is released to provide energy.**

Fig. 3

When we are starving or need energy this cascade occurs.

Pancreas releases glucagon → converts glycogen back into glucose or

breaks down fat for energy.

The body's first priority after it eats is to fill the liver glycogen stores first, which have a capacity of about 100 grams. The muscles are next, and have a capacity of around 250-400g. After the muscles are full is when we need to be careful. **Any food consumed after this will be shuttled, with the help of insulin, to fat cells for storage.** Not at all what we want. So the trick is to consume just enough carbohydrates, at the appropriate times, to make sure we don't store them as fat. When we need energy again, all our body has to do is release glucagon, which initiates the breakdown of glycogen, and thus provides energy in the form of glucose.

The breakdown of glycogen *back* into glucose is called **glycogenolysis,** and the breakdown of fat is called **lipolysis.** As long as there is glycogen or fat present in the body, they can be converted into usable sources of energy to keep us functioning.

When is Insulin a Good Thing?

What if we don't eat, don't supply the body with any nutrients, what happens then? Well, the body won't call a draw and just stand still. It will still release glucagon as blood sugar levels fall, and once all the glycogen is depleted, our body will begin to break down muscle and fat to produce glucose through another process called **gluconeogenesis**. Gluconeogenesis is the generation of glucose from non-carbohydrate sources, such as muscle tissue and fat, and is exactly what occurs when glycogen levels run low. **The body has various survival tactics and this is one of them.** While breaking down fat is a good thing, the loss of muscle makes this situation unacceptable.

The bad news doesn't stop there. The body also releases an unfriendly hormone called cortisol. **Cortisol** is known as the stress hormone, the body releases it in times of severe stress, poor nutrition, or sickness. It absolutely is a hormone you never want to see. The good news is that insulin opposes cortisol release, so by consuming healthy carbohydrate sources at the appropriate times, we can prevent this hormone from arising. Not only that, but after working out, be it cardio or lifting, the body is in a very fragile state. It has used all its energy reserves in the form of glucose and glycogen to get us through the workout.

Now is the time when insulin is an absolute must. The insulin released with the consumption of a post-workout meal will create a vacuum effect. Rather than being stored as fat *the muscles and liver will absorb the nutrients,* which remember, is priority number #1! We will discuss this in more detail in the chapters to come, but for now, realize that **consuming foods that spike insulin levels is never more important than after a workout.**

Is Insulin Ever a Bad Thing?

Now, it's not all-good news for insulin, as there are times when you don't want an insulin spike. These times happen to be when you already have full glycogen stores, or anytime you are trying to burn fat. *We want insulin to be non-existent at these times.* **The body shuts fat loss down and initiates the uptake of nutrients anytime insulin is present.** So, if you have full glycogen stores, an insulin release will shuttle nutrients into fat cells, as the liver and muscles are already full. If you are trying to burn fat and insulin is released, the body will terminate fat loss and initiate storage. That is why it is frustrating to see people doing cardio in the morning while drinking Gatorade, orange juice or a fruity drink. Insulin is being produced with each swallow and fat burning stops. The sad thing is, most don't know it, and will continue to drink these beverages while seeing few gains.

So now we know that if glycogen is already stored in great amounts, or if insulin is present in the blood, the body will not burn much fat. In fact, if insulin is present it most likely will cause the storage of more fat! After all it is a "storage" hormone. Anytime we exercise our body's first reaction is to use stored glycogen or glucose in our bloodstream. However, what if you exercised when very little glycogen was left, and no glucose or insulin was present at all? Say, first thing in the morning after not eating all night? You would burn fat like crazy!

Whoa! I thought you just said we would burn up muscle if we didn't eat? I did in fact say that, but there is a trick, and I'll tell you all about it later. The key at this point is to understand the power of exercise, specifically cardiovascular training in the morning before breakfast. You see, during an 8-hour fast while sleeping, the body just doesn't stop working, it uses the stored glycogen from the previous day to keep the engine running at night. While liver glycogen stores will supply energy throughout the night, the muscles aren't as cooperative, and will only use their stored glycogen during resistance training. That is why lifting weights is so important, not only will it initiate muscle glycogen use during your workout, but it will further deplete the overall glycogen stores, making it easier to tap into fat stores when you exercise. As you read this book, you will further realize how you can manipulate insulin to gain muscle and lose fat. If we understand the physiology behind this potent hormone, we can use it to achieve our goals.

Growth Hormone

Anytime the term **growth hormone (GH)** is brought up, all you seem to hear is,"I don't use steroids," or "I am all natural." What we fail to realize is that we all produce a great deal of growth hormone naturally, and that it can be manipulated to burn fat and build muscle.

The Basics of GH

GH is produced in the **pituitary gland** before traveling to the muscles, liver, and fat cells. Once there, it performs various functions, one of which is initiating the cascade that leads to muscular growth. How? Well, the release of GH produces another protein, **Insulin-like growth factor 1 (IGF-1)**, a key ingredient to muscular gains and fat loss. Once GH reaches the liver, which remember is one of its destination sites, IGF-1 is produced. Once the production of IGF-1 is complete, it travels to the muscle were it initiates growth. So as you are starting to see, GH production starts a chain of reactions that all lead to increased muscular gains and fat metabolism (Fig 4).

Fig. 4

Pituitary Gland produces GH →   GH travels to liver →   IGF-1

produced → IGF-1 travels to muscles →   Muscle Growth/Fat Loss is

the result!

Natural GH Production

There are two major producers of GH and one is a good nights sleep. That's right, get a solid nights rest and you will produce more GH. Lactic acid, which is produced during intense bouts of exercise, is however the major catalyst to GH production. The "burn" we feel while exercising signifies that glycogen is being used and lactic acid is being produced. In fact, studies have shown that those who engage in short rest periods and intense training sessions produce far greater amounts of GH than those who don't train intensely and take longer rest periods. The reason is simply because the body produces far more lactic acid with shorter rest periods, and thus, more GH.

The Results Are Seen Later

It is important to note, that numerous studies have shown the greatest effects of GH are not seen until hours after your workout. Knowing that, it's no coincidence that intense cardio or lifting sessions cause the greatest increase in GH hours after you train. This is just one of the reasons I favor high intensity training, which refers to workouts of increased intensity and shorter duration. This prolonged fat burning effect can make your training more efficient, as even after you have showered and are taking it easy, GH continues to burn fat at a remarkable pace!

GH and Insulin: Friends or Foes?

An interesting point to GH production is its inhibition by insulin. Therefore, **GH has is greatest effect without tremendous amounts of insulin present** (Fig. 5). What this means is that you will produce the greatest amount of GH on an empty stomach or with a minimal amount of glucose flowing through your bloodstream. Hence, insulin release will be very low and the effects of GH will be maximized. The problem is, insulin is needed to cause an influx of nutrients into muscles following a workout. Once you eat sugary carbohydrates post-workout, you will usher a massive insulin spike, thus slowing down GH production and fat loss. It seems contradictory that both are so important to muscle growth, but inhibit each other in regards to fat loss. That is why many find it difficult to gain muscle *and* lose fat. I promise though, it can be done. The key is understanding how to use both to maximize our gains.

Fig. 5

Fat Loss Scenario	Muscle Gain Scenario
Workout→GH→Fat Loss	Workout→GH→Muscle
or	or
Workout+Insulin→GH→Fat Loss	Workout+Insulin+GH→Muscle

Summary:

1. Short rest periods and intense training causes the most GH production secondary to the production of lactic acid.
2. Growth hormone production is highest, and promotes maximum fat loss, when low insulin levels are present.
3. Although insulin inhibits fat loss, it is extremely important in regards to recovery and muscle growth.

Therefore, to maximize the production and positive effects of both, we must cater our training to each hormone. We should perform cardio on an empty stomach or hours after our last meal. Therefore, we can maximize GH and fat loss, as insulin levels will be greatly reduced. After lifting, one should consume a post workout drink to initiate an insulin spike and begin the repair process. Although reduced, GH will still be present to aid in muscular growth, along with testosterone if you have trained hard enough. If you do these things, you will have a great balance between muscular gains and fat loss. It all has to do with knowledge and nutrient timing.

As you will see later in this book, consuming specific nutrients before, during, and after training is vital to maximum fat loss, muscle protection, and gains. Training hard will allow more GH production to aid in fat loss, but you'll get the anabolic effects of insulin with the proper consumption of specific nutrients. While it is very difficult to build muscle while burning substantial amounts of fat, it can be done, just at a reduced rate.

Does It Work?

In preparation for a bodybuilding show in 2006, I did cardio every morning, ate one hour before my lifting sessions, consumed specific "workout" drinks while training, and used high intensity training techniques. The intense training and proper diet increased my testosterone and GH production, while morning cardio on an empty stomach maxed out my fat loss. Consuming my workout drinks, during and immediately after training, allowed for sufficient insulin release to maximize recovery. Later in this book, I'll describe the exact nutrition and supplement protocols that allowed me to gain muscle while reducing my body fat to 5% for the contest.

Why Does Insulin Inhibit Fat Loss?

Why does insulin stop fat loss in its tracks? One of the major reasons is the inhibition of GH, but the other is **hormone sensitive lipase (HSL)**. HSL is yet another vital component to losing body fat. Its ability to aid in fat loss is accentuated by GH and glucagon, while inhibited by insulin. Another point of interest is that insulin not only inhibits HSL, but promotes the opposite, **lipoprotein lipase (LPL)**. The negative attribute of LPL, much like insulin, is that it aids in fat storage (Fig. 6). The benefit of HSL is that it breaks down fat cells into individual components called fatty acids, and sends them into the bloodstream. From there, they will be transported to various cells and used as fuel.

Fig. 6

1) GH promotes→HSL→ Results in Increased Fat Burning

2) Insulin promotes→ LPL→Results in Decreased Fat Burning

In summary, all we need to understand are a couple basic facts.

1. If we want to burn the most fat, we must inhibit insulin and promote GH.

2. We must also realize that the consumption of foods that promote insulin release is vital post-workout to initiate recovery and growth.

You must have a basic understanding of hormone functions to properly set up your training and nutrition programs.

Summary

+   **Testosterone** is produced in the testes or ovaries, and is responsible for the physical characteristics of males and females, as well as affecting sex drive. It is a potent muscle builder, which is why men produce more than females. Maximize testosterone production by consuming marginal amounts of cholesterol and saturated fat, training hard, and never letting your daily fat consumption dip below 10%. Obesity, lack of sleep, and over-training all decrease testosterone.

- **Cholesterol** is a necessity for testosterone production and other cell processes. It can be consumed as cholesterol, but can also be synthesized in the liver with the consumption of saturated fats from egg yolks and red meats.

- **Low- Density Lipoprotein (LDL)** is generally thought of as the "bad" cholesterol but is a precursor to the formation of testosterone. It acts as a "carrier" of cholesterol so that it can be transported around the body to perform various tasks. As an example, it "drops" cholesterol off at the testes so that it can begin the synthesis of testosterone.

- **High-Density Lipoprotein (HDL)** is generally thought of as the "good" cholesterol and is responsible for clearing the blood of excess cholesterol. It basically "picks-up" the excess cholesterol and transports it back to the liver so it can be excreted.

- **Insulin** is released by the beta cells of the pancreas after we consume food, specifically carbohydrates, and essentially stops fat loss in its tracks. It is a storage hormone and initiates the uptake of glucose into our muscles and liver to be stored as glycogen. If the liver and muscles reach maximum storage capacity, then the liver will convert excess glucose into fat and transport them to fat cells via LDL. Insulin is essential following a workout to promote the uptake of nutrients and initiate the rebuilding process. Limit insulin to increase fat burning. Increase insulin to promote muscle gains. Timing is everything.

- **Glucagon** is released by the alpha cells of the pancreas when blood sugar levels are low. This often occurs when we haven't eaten for a significant amount of time. It is essentially the opposite of insulin, and promotes the breakdown of glycogen into glucose, as well as the breakdown of muscle and fat. Glucagon is released to provide the body with energy.

- **Cortisol** is known as the stress hormone. It is opposed by insulin and will destroy your muscular gains and fat loss. It is present in any catabolic environment and should be avoided at all costs. Consuming a "workout" drink during and after weight training can severely derail the production of cortisol. Lack of sleep, poor diet, and over-training also contribute to its production.

- **Growth hormone** is a major proponent of fat loss and muscle gains. It is produced at an accelerated rate when lactic acid is present, and is reduced in the presence of insulin. To maximize output and fat loss, train intensely while minimizing insulin release. While GH and fat-loss are maximized with low insulin output, we must find a middle ground, as muscle gains and preservation are also a priority. Using intense training protocols and consuming proper nutrients can allow GH, testosterone, and insulin to have a synergistic action in regards to muscle gains. Although GH and insulin oppose each other in relation to fat loss, they work together to build muscle and inhibit cortisol.

- **Insulin-Like Growth Factor-1 (IGF-1)** is produced when GH reaches the liver. It is vital to the synthesis of new muscle. Produce GH and you will produce IGF-1.

- **Hormone sensitive lipase (HSL)** is a major player in the breakdown of fat before it can be used as fuel.

- **Lipoprotein lipase (LPL)** is a major player in the storage of body fat.

Definitions and Key Points:

**Carbohydrates, Fats and Protein are all sources of energy because they can be converted via various processes to adenosine tri-phosphate (ATP) in the body. Carbohydrates are the best at doing this.*

Glycogenolysis: breakdown of glycogen back into glucose.

Gluconeogenesis: formation of glucose from non-carbohydrate sources.

Lipolysis: breakdown of fat for energy.

Chapter 3

THE MACRONUTRIENTS- CARBOHYDRATES/ PROTEIN/FATS

Now we have a solid knowledge base in regards to our hormone profiles. The next step is to truly understand the foods we eat and how they affect us. Once you read this section, you'll have a thorough understanding of how nutrients can help you attain the physique you desire.

The Purpose of Carbohydrates

In our discussion of the macronutrients, which include protein, fats and carbohydrates, we will begin with the later. Carbohydrates are classified as a macronutrient, and when broken down to their simplest form, glucose, provide one of two things.

Carbohydrates can:

1. Provide fuel for us in the form of blood glucose and eventual ATP production.

2. Be stored in the muscle and liver as glycogen, or as fat in fat cells.

Insulin, as you now know, is responsible for shuttling glucose into our muscles and liver, so that it can be stored as glycogen. Again, the muscles are able to hold around 250-400 g of glycogen, and the liver can hold approximately 100 grams. Once these stores are full, and our energy needs have been met, any excess carbohydrates will be converted to fat. This is why carbohydrates are the macronutrient most responsible for unwanted fat accumulation.

Without a doubt, eating carbohydrates is necessary for proper brain function and energy, as well as keeping us from having frequent mood swings. In fact, low carbohydrate diets have been associated with depression, low sex drive, fatigue, irritability, and rapid weight fluctuations. So how do we use carbohydrates to aid in the pursuit of our goals? Through a basic understanding of how they differ, and when we should consume them.

The Basics of Carbohydrates

Carbohydrates are one of the quickest sources of energy at our disposal. **Each gram of carbohydrate yields 4 calories.** Essentially, if you consume 50 g of carbohydrates, you would be taking in 200 calories (50g x 4 cal/g=200 calories). Carbohydrates all cause a release of insulin, but the rate at which this happens differs with the type of carbohydrate you consume. Carbohydrates should be thought of as **complex**, which are slow digesting, and **simple**, which are quick to digest. The faster the digestion, the more insulin will be released (Fig 7). Complex carbohydrates include breads, pasta, oatmeal, rice, and beans. Simple carbohydrates include sugars, sports drinks, honey, and juices. There are also **fibrous** carbohydrates such as vegetables. While they are complex by nature, I consider them fibrous as you can eat nearly as many as you want and not worry about gaining weight. Vegetables are extremely slow to digest and cause a very minimal release of insulin, which is why they are so healthy and filling.

Fig. 7

Complex Carbohydrates→slower to digest→lower insulin release

Simple Carbohydrates→faster to digest→greater insulin release

Fruit and Milk

While having characteristics of simple, fibrous, and complex carbohydrates, fruit is one of the healthiest foods we can consume. Fruit has a great deal of fiber, which slows digestion, as well as beneficial vitamins and minerals. Fruit however contains a type of sugar called fructose, and thus earns the classification as a simple carbohydrate. Milk is another healthy food that actually has simple carbohydrates in the form of lactose, or "milk sugar." It is also filled with calcium for bone health and protein to rebuild muscles. Milk contains a combination of simple sugars in glucose and galactose, which together make up lactose.

Despite fruit and milk not creating as severe of an insulin spike as glucose by itself, it does so nonetheless. Although I believe we should all consume fruit and milk products to benefit our physiques and overall health, they should be excluded, or eaten at specific times, if one wishes to lose body fat very quickly.

Why Can Fruit And Milk Be A Problem?

One reason fruit can be a problem deals with its poor muscle absorption post workout. Not only is it slower to digest than other simple carbohydrates, but also contains fructose, the type of sugar found in fruit. Fructose is unable to be stored as muscle glycogen, and can only be stored in the liver. Once the 100 g maximum of liver glycogen has been met, **then** the liver will convert any excess fructose into blood-glucose and/or body fat. Our goal is to re-fill our muscle glycogen stores **as quickly as possible post-workout**, thus making fruit a poor choice.

Although you can't refill your muscles glycogen using fruit post workout, it is still a good pre-workout carbohydrate source. Fruit is slow to digest, and will provide an energy source once converted to glucose in the liver. What about milk? Milk again contains lactose, which is a sugar, and therefore can spike insulin. Not only that, but it must be broken down into glucose, and that can cause a problem as many are lactose intolerant and can't complete this conversion. Although I love milk, when trying to get very lean, I have noticed that I won't lose body fat as rapidly if I don't consume it at very specific times. This again is secondary to the sugar content of milk and ensuing insulin spike. Recent studies have shown that those on low calorie diets who consume milk products actually notice an increase in fat metabolism. Other studies have shown no difference. Each individual varies and therefore you must experiment to see where you stand.

So When Can I Consume Fruit and Milk?

While many steer clear of fruit and milk all together when trying to get very lean, others do not, and find great success. *The secret is nutrient timing.* The key is to consume them, as well as most carbohydrates, at a time of day when they are more likely to be used as energy and not fat gain. These periods include *breakfast, mid-morning, and surrounding your workout.* If you do this, you can still benefit from fruit and milk, while not slowing down your transformation. Should you consume fruit, it is best to focus on apples, bananas, oranges and berries. These have lower GI scores than pineapples or mangos and therefore keep sugar more stable. If at all possible, limit the amount of *dried fruit* you consume. The dried forms of any fruit, such as raisins, are much higher in calories and sugar than their natural or frozen counterparts.

The Glycemic Index

The glycemic index (GI) is something you must understand to create an effective nutrition program. This index refers to how quickly a food is broken down, in comparison to pure glucose with a score of 100, and converted to glucose in the blood. Obviously, the more glucose released, the higher the ensuing insulin spike. So, lower GI scores promote less insulin release and more stable blood sugars.

GI scores are **lower for complex carbohydrates and higher for simple carbohydrates**. The higher the glycemic index, the quicker the digestion, glucose release, and ensuing insulin spike. This can quickly lead to fat accumulation. Not only that, but eating carbohydrates high on the glycemic index makes us even hungrier! How? Well, the food is so rapidly digested and processed, the body goes from a high blood sugar to a low one very quickly, as the sudden rush of insulin quickly removes all blood sugar.

The body then desires more food, not to mention making your moody and lethargic. So what do we do? We eat more and more, which quickly leads to less muscle and more fat gains.

Think about it, the last time you ate two cookies, did you want more? In contrast, the last time you ate a huge bowl of oatmeal, what then? The fact that you probably wanted a few more cookies but couldn't wait to be done with your big bowl of oatmeal proves my point. The reason is that the cookies, or any sugary food, are high on the GI scale and will spike insulin quickly. Oatmeal, high fiber wheat bread, brown rice, sweet potatoes, and black beans are all low GI and will therefore cause a slow, steady release of glucose, resulting in a slower release of insulin. We also can't forget that fiber, which is higher in complex carbohydrates, slows digestion immensely. Vegetables have one of the highest fiber contents of all foods. When was the last time you wanted three bowls of those things? Even fruit, containing the simple sugar fructose, is lower on the GI scale than glucose, despite both being simple sugars. While not ALWAYS true:

- Complex Carbohydrates tend to be Lower on the GI scale
- Simple Carbohydrates tend to be Higher on the GI scale

Now remember from our discussion on insulin, the more dramatic the insulin release, the harder it is to burn fat, and the easier it is to store it. The end result of eating low GI carbohydrates then is the slow release of glucose for energy. **The slower the release of glucose, the slower the release of insulin**. This keeps you full for a prolonged period of time and makes it difficult for the body to store fat.

The Key to The Puzzle

The key is to use the body's natural physiology to our advantage. We talked about the body using glucose and glycogen (a.k.a stored glucose) as its primary energy source during exercise. While you lift weights or exercise, the body is slowly using glucose and breaking down glycogen as fuel. In fact, if you do cardio, right after lifting, you will tap right into your fat stores, as the body has used most of its glycogen and glucose to get you through the workout. Our body needs fuel to keep going so it must start burning fat. It is the second best time, next to early morning cardio on an empty stomach, to significantly burn fat.

So why not work out and not eat for hours, surely your body will keep burning fat? Well, not so fast. After the completion of your workout, you have a maximum of one hour to consume a post workout meal, or your body will switch gears on you. It will continue to release cortisol, which burns muscle for fuel, shuts down fat loss, and hampers your immune system. After you have completed your workout, with all your depleted glycogen, the body is begging for nutrients. That's why **the post exercise meal is by far the most important of the day.** I'll say that again, the most important of the day. Now is the time to eat high GI carbohydrates and a fast acting protein. This will cause a large insulin spike and reverse the process back into an anabolic state.

One more time....Why Do I Want A Massive Insulin Spike?

You want the insulin to shuttle all your nutrients back into your muscle to initiate repair, and negate any negative side effects the stress of the workout might have had. The body will have a difficult time storing fat at this time as it's first priority is to refill the liver and muscle glycogen stores. The high GI carbohydrates, causing a massive insulin spike, will shuttle all the nutrients you consume into your liver and muscles, making it very difficult to store fat. Now, don't get too excited, there is a limit, and if you eat too much of anything, even plain chicken breasts and rice cakes, you will gain fat.

The best choices post-workout include **fast acting protein and simple GI carbohydrates, which include Gatorade, juice, jelly, and honey.** Even white bread, although being a complex carbohydrate, has a high GI score, and is acceptable post workout. In the coming chapters I'll show you the protocol I use in the hours surrounding my workout . This nutrition protocol will replenish all your glycogen stores, limit fat uptake, and quickly initiate muscle repair. The only foods to shy away from post workout are low GI/high fiber foods, such as vegetables, and any type of fat. Both of these foods will dramatically slow digestion, which is the opposite of what you want at this time.

Summary

+ **Complex and Fibrous Carbohydrates (usually low GI and high fiber)**
+ Slow digestion and insulin release.
+ Should never be consumed post workout.
+ Ideal at all other meals as they slow digestion, minimize fat gain, and maintain a feeling of fullness.

Complex and Fibrous Carbohydrate Sources (usually low GI)

1. Oatmeal

2. Whole Wheat or Ezekiel Bread

3. Sweet Potatoes

4. Brown Rice

5. Vegetables

Simple Carbohydrate (usually high GI)

+ Cause massive insulin spike and fat storage if used at the wrong time
+ Always consume post workout- but can also be consumed at breakfast-both times when the body is low on glycogen and blood sugar.
+ When eaten at the wrong time of day, one of the main reasons individuals gain body fat.
+ Fruit and milk, although healthy, can make it difficult to burn body

fat secondary to the simple carbohydrates they contain. The key is to time your intake of fruits and milk.

- Stay away from fruit post-workout, as the muscles will not be able to refill glycogen stores with fructose-the sugar found in fruit.

- If you consume fruit, focus more on natural or frozen varieties rather than dried. This will keep calories and sugar intake much lower.

- Apples, bananas, oranges and berries have lower GI scores than mangos or pineapple.

Simple Carbohydrate Sources (usually High GI):

1. Gatorade

2. Jelly

3. Honey

4. Fruit Juice

5. Fruit (lower GI than most all simple carbohydrates)

6. Milk

Protein

The word protein comes from the Greek word, *Proteous*, which means, "of first importance." Nothing could be further from the truth. Understanding carbohydrates is key to making sure we limit fat gains and have energy to workout. However, without protein, forget building muscle or keeping it for that matter. Even vegetarians need protein to survive. Another benefit of protein is that it is much harder to eat a surplus than it is carbohydrates. This is because the stomach releases a **protein called YY** that significantly reduces our appetite when we consume meals high in protein. That is why you are less likely to eat ten chicken breasts than ten chocolate chip cookies.

Protein is also very thermogenic, meaning it actually causes the body to burn more calories during digestion than either carbohydrates or fat!

Now, in regards to repair and growth, no macronutrient is more important that protein. If you exercise and are deficient in the amount of protein you consume, you will never attain the physique you desire. Protein, like carbohydrates, is a macronutrient. Similar to carbohydrates, **it yields 4 calories per gram.** Protein, once consumed, is broken down into micronutrients called amino acids, with its primary role being muscle repair. Amino acids are what make up protein, and protein is what makes up muscle.

There are twenty amino acids, eleven of them being non-essential, or made by the body. Non-essential simply means we do not need to consume them to have adequate amounts in our body. That doesn't mean that we can't take in more to enhance the effects. One such example is **glutamine**, the most important non-essential amino acids for athletes, and the most prolific in skeletal muscle. We will discuss this amino acid in more detail in the chapter on supplements, but it is vital to say the least. It aids in immunity, muscle repair, and energy production to name a few of its benefits. That leaves nine as essential, which simply means we must consume them in the food we eat to make sure we obtain adequate amounts.

Of the nine essential amino acids, three make up what we call the **branch chain amino acids (BCAA)**. The BCAA consist of leucine, isoleucine and valine. Leucine is the most anabolic, or muscle building, of all the amino acids and is the first to initiate repair in muscles after a workout. The BCAA are also the first to be used as fuel if the body should have to break down muscle in the absence of nutrients. In fact, they are often used to synthesize more glutamine, which again can aid in repair, immunity, and energy production. Remember that muscle breakdown, or catabolism, is what happens if you don't eat immediately following a workout. Therefore, *if you consume BCAA before, during, and after a training session, they not only are present to provide fuel, but they are already starting the repair process while we are working out.* We will hit more on that later, but I want you to realize how important BCAA and glutamine are to our overall success.

The Basics of Protein

The primary source of protein is animal meat, such as chicken, beef, lamb and turkey. Protein is also found in fish, eggs, dairy products and nuts. Protein supplements are also an option, and one that should constitute the protein you consume post workout. The reason is its fast acting quality, and ability to get to the muscles quickly and efficiently. As far as your other meals, you should consume a variety of protein sources and spread them out throughout the day. How much do we need? In my opinion, for an athlete who trains and damages muscle tissue, **1 gram, per pound of bodyweight, per day, is ideal**. Many, including myself, consume a little more, but 1 g/lbs/day is a good place to start.

Now, there are lean protein sources and fatty protein sources. As an individual who is trying to obtain the leanest and most muscular physique possible, lean protein should make up the bulk of your diet. Don't be fooled into thinking that fatty protein is bad though. There is a time and place to consume them. As an example, I believe you should occasionally eat red meat and egg yolks, which contain saturated fat, and aid in hormone production and muscle building. I prefer venison, buffalo, and lean beef, as it minimizes the amount of saturated fat, while still providing its benefits. Omega-3 fatty acids, found in salmon for example, also have their benefits. We'll describe more on fat in the next section but know that fatty proteins, as well as lean sources, have their place.

It is rare for any food to be composed solely of fat, carbohydrates, or protein. They are however usually dominated by one; with another macronutrient present in smaller amounts. In the case of protein, it is always protein and fat, never carbohydrates, unless the protein source has something added to it. Ideally, you should eat fatty protein in the absence of carbohydrates, as fat and carbohydrates are both sources of energy. That means, if you have salmon or steak, you shouldn't include a potato or oatmeal, as your fuel source comes from the fat in the meat. Excess energy, either carbohydrates or fat, will do nothing more than add body fat. If you eat chicken breasts or grilled white fish, you can consume carbohydrates or fat with your meal, as these protein sources have little energy. These simple facts can make sure you get the nutrients you need at the correct times without gaining excess fat.

Now that we have discussed the whole food sources of protein, lets discuss the supplemented forms found in liquid and powdered varieties. They can be confusing, but I'll try to simplify it here. It is vital to know this information or you could buy the wrong type. I use supplemental forms of protein often, as I can't eat that much whole food protein and don't have time to cook it all. Using supplemented forms can add ease to your life, and are actually more beneficial in certain situations.

Now, there are **four types** of protein supplements that you may be familiar with, although they are found in natural food as well. All you really need to know about each are the basics. I have listed them below in order of importance. Most proteins available today, whether whole food, liquid, or powder, contain a percentage of some or all of those listed. Knowing what each does can make your choices easier.

1. **Whey**

2. **Casein**

3. **Soy**

4. **Egg**

Whey- By far the most important post-workout as it digests rapidly. This type of protein has the highest concentration of glutamine and BCAA's, which again include leucine, isoleucine, and valine. BCAA and glutamine, again, are important because they initiate the muscle repair process, aid in immunity, energy production, and protect against muscle wasting. There are various forms of whey such as:

+ *Whey protein hydrosylate-*already broken down into amino acids. Can be expensive but absorbs very rapidly.

- *Whey protein isolate*-pure form of whey with almost all lactose removed.

- *Whey protein concentrate*-most common and is inexpensive. Used to contain high amounts of lactose but now many products have it removed.

Important Pearl: the consumption of whey protein will not prevent muscle breakdown as efficiently if there is insufficient amounts of BCAA and glutamine present in each serving. While whey does a tremendous job of initiating repair after working out, adequate BCAA and glutamine concentrations are much more efficient at inhibiting muscle breakdown. Not only that, but they significantly enhance the muscle repair and growth process. If these amino acids are present, as in most high quality whey sold today, the combination will maximize **protection and repair.** That is why you shouldn't buy the cheapest whey you can find, as it often lacks sufficient amounts of these critical amino acids.

You need at least 5g of BCAA and glutamine, and more is recommended, to protect from muscle wasting, so check to see how much is included per serving. I personally consume a separate serving of BCAA and glutamine 15 minutes prior to drinking my whey shake, to make sure I get an adequate amount of each. Also, the absorption is much better when consumed by themselves, opposed to mixed in with your whey. So, should you decide to consume a separate mix in addition to your whey, take it 15-30 minutes before your whey shake as the absorption will be better. We will discuss more on this topic in the chapter on supplements.

*As a side note, when you hear the word whey, it almost always is in reference to a powder or liquid supplement, perfect for post workout because it digests rapidly. However, it can be found in natural foods such as milk, in which 20% of its composition is whey.

Casein- this form of protein is **very slow digesting** and the best to take before bed. Some recent studies have shown that a combination of whey and casein is best post workout. The reason is that the whey will initiate **immediate** repair, and the casein will allow a **continuous, long lasting**

supply of amino acids. Milk products (milk, cheese, cottage cheese etc) are 80% casein protein and 20% whey.

Important Pearl: casein will do little to **_quickly_** initiate repair, as it is slow acting. On the other hand, it is very valuable in regards to protecting against muscle breakdown at night and between meals, secondary to its slow release characteristics.

Soy-this protein has been talked down on for years as it was believed to cause estrogen like effects in those who took it. It is found most readily in plants, as well as in supplement form. **It is second only to whey in its ability to be absorbed quickly.** I personally don't use soy, but more studies are showing that it does have value. The one thing it does have over the others is the **highest concentration of arginine.** This amino acid is linked to blood vessel dilation and the basis of many pre-workout drinks revolves around arginine.

Egg Protein- second only to soy in arginine content, but almost as slow to digest as casein. That basically means it can be used at bedtime to ensure a longer amino acid release, although not as prolonged as casein. It can also be used post workout, with the knowledge that it won't be absorbed as quickly as whey or soy.

The bottom line: I ideally choose protein powders that contain percentages of whey, casein, and egg. I have not used much soy, but that doesn't mean it isn't a good source. I like to make sure at least 50% of my protein consumption comes from whole foods such as meat, fish, eggs, and dairy. I use powdered protein 100% of the time post workout, and again like a combination of whey, egg, and casein. Now that you know what to look for, you can make better decisions based on your goals.

Summary

- Protein is vital for muscle protection and repair.
- You should consume at least 1 g of protein, per pound of body weight, per day.

- Glutamine is the most important **non-essential** amino acid. It aids in immunity, repair, and energy production to name a few of its benefits.
- The BCAA are the most important **essential** amino acids in regards to inhibiting muscle breakdown and initiating repair.
- Leucine is the most important **individual** amino acid in regards to *repair and muscle growth*.
- Glutamine is the most important **individual** amino acid in regards to *immunity*.
- Whey protein is the fastest absorbed protein.
- Casein is a slowest released protein, which provides the body amino acids for hours after consumption.
- Egg is not digested as quickly as whey or as slowly as casein.
- Post workout, consuming a BCAA/glutamine drink mix 15-30 minutes before your protein shake is ideal to maximize absorption.
- A combination of whey, casein, and egg protein makes up the perfect post-workout shake. Don't forget to add your high GI-simple carbohydrates source!
- Fatty protein has its place for hormone production.
- If you eat fatty protein, don't consume carbohydrates other than vegetables with your meal.
- If you eat lean protein, you can consume complex carbohydrates or fat to aid in slowing digestion and energy. Try to avoid eating fat and carbohydrates together. This will eventually lead to fat gain.

	Lean Protein Sources	**Fatty Protein Sources**
1.	Chicken Breast	Chicken Thigh or Leg
2.	Turkey Breast	Turkey Thigh or Leg
3.	White Fish/Tuna	Salmon
4.	Egg Whites	Whole Egg
5.	Venison	Beef Steak
6.	Protein Supplements	Nuts
7.	Cottage Cheese/Skim Milk	Lamb

Fat

Fat. Of all the macronutrients, it is the most misunderstood. In fact, this entire country has made billions of dollars on "fat-free" food. So, I am here to tell you that this marketing scheme is one of the main reasons we have a higher percentage of obese Americans than ever! Why is "fat-free" bad? Well, nothing in life is free, so to compensate for the bland taste that removing fat does to a food, sugar is added. After reading the segment on insulin and carbohydrates, I think you now understand why it's a major cause of increasing body fat. Remember, once we spike our insulin levels the uptake of nutrients begins. However, if the glycogen tanks are already filled, it has to go somewhere, and that place is usually fat cells.

The Basics of Fat

Fat, scientifically referred to as triglycerides, are essential made up of three fatty acids with a glycerol backbone. When fat is used as energy by the body, it first must be separated from its glycerol backbone by HSL. It is then sent via the bloodstream to the mitochondria of various organ cells, which will use it for energy.

Fat is also the most calorie dense macronutrient, yielding 9 calories per gram. This is over two times what a similar amount of carbohydrates or protein would provide! Without a doubt, overeating this macronutrient can definitely lead to a poor looking physique. Yet, despite these qualities, **it is extremely important to consume fat in your diet.** Healthy fats are essential for hormone production, cardiovascular health, and reducing inflammation. Fats can also slow digestion, making you feel full longer. In fact, adequate consumption of the "healthy" fats will actually promote fat loss!

Without a portion of your caloric intake coming from these essential fats, it will be difficult to burn fat and obtain the physique you want. This is because the body needs these fats to produce the hormones so vital to increasing your metabolism and building muscle. In so doing, it is more likely to use excess fat as fuel to keep us going. If you take in too little fat, or none at all, the body may panic and hold onto fat rather than burn it. Essentially, you need fat to survive, and not incorporating an adequate amount of healthy fat into your diet will worsen your physique.

10-20% of your daily caloric intake should be composed off healthy fats. **The only time to avoid the consumption of fat is post workout, and any meal in which carbohydrates are involved.** The reason to avoid them post workout is that fats delay absorption. Although it would keep you full longer, post workout is the last time you would want an effect such as this. Likewise, you would never want to combine fats with carbohydrates, as they both serve as energy sources. Combining fat with protein or protein with carbohydrates is fine, but try to refrain from eating fats and carbohydrates in the same meal. This will usually lead to fat gain. The key is to select foods with a moderate amount of healthy fats to benefit your physique and health, rather than hinder it.

Now that we have a better understanding of how beneficial fat can be, what exactly constitutes "healthy" fat? There are two categories of fat that are most commonly referred to. These are **saturated and unsaturated fats.** Saturated fats are found in foods such as cheese, red meat, and egg yolks, and **should be limited in the amount you consume.** I do believe they should not be excluded though, as red meat contains high amounts of protein, vitamins, and some creatine. As we discussed earlier, saturated fat from red meat and egg yolks can also aid in testosterone production. I limit my saturated fat intake to lean red meats and egg yolks, trying to eat them only 2-3 times per week.

Now, the "good" fats are unsaturated, and consist of **monounsaturated and polyunsaturated fats.** Some examples of monounsaturated fats are peanut butter, almonds, olive oil, and sesame seeds. Polyunsaturated fats are more important in regards to health and physical transformation, and include the "essential" fatty acids (EFA), omega-3 and omega-6. The EFA's are deemed "essential" as we must obtain them through outside food sources.

Omega-3 fatty acids include **eicosapentaenoic acid (EPA) and docosahexaenoic acid (DHA)** found in cold water fish and fish oil supplements, along with **alpha-linolenic acid (ALA),** found in walnuts and flax seed oil. Omega-6 fatty acids or linoleic acid, are found in sunflower and vegetable oil. Over all, the omega-3 fatty acids, specifically eicosapentaenoic acid (EPA) and docosahexaenoic acid (DHA), are of the greatest benefit and the type of fat you should focus on the most. Omega-6 fatty acids have a very small role in promoting our health and are not nearly as important as the omega-3's.

You may already be familiar with omega-3 fatty acids, as they are one of the most talked about supplements in the media today. While you can find them in cold water fish, walnuts, flax seed oil and supplements, *you must focus on the source that provides the most EPA and DHA.* **In saying that, the best sources come from the consumption of cold-water fish such as salmon and tuna, or actually consuming fish oil capsules.** These sources contain the highest concentration of EPA and DHA. I supplement with 3-4g of fish oil capsules per day, while eating fish a few times per week. Walnuts and flax seed oil, while both being sources of omega-3 fatty acids, provide only a small amount of EPA/DHA once metabolized.

Aren't They All The Same?

Despite all omega-3 fatty acids being healthy, fish and fish oil supplements have the highest concentration of EPA/DHA. Walnuts and flax seed oil, containing alpha-linolenic acid, a type of omega-3, must convert to EPA/ DHA, and this often leads to poor output. Therefore, you would have to consume far more walnuts or flax seed oil to equal what you might obtain from fish and fish oil supplements. Remember, it is not necessarily the omega-3 fatty acids that are so beneficial, but their metabolized end products, namely eicosapentaenoic acid (EPA) and docosahexaenoic acid (DHA). The higher the concentrations of these end products, the greater the benefit.

CLA

The only other fat I'll briefly describe is **Conjugated Linoleic acid (CLA)**. It is an isomer of linoleic acids, and is found in the meat and dairy products of ruminants such as cows. It is actually a trans-fat, although nothing like the negative trans-fat associated with French fries and potato chips. Supplementing with 3 grams of CLA per day can aid in fat loss by inhibiting the uptake and storage of fat after meals. It actually prevents fat cells from growing larger! More and more research of late is supporting the benefits of this supplement, and I have found great success using it. Although it is found in dairy and beef products, it is far more advantageous to consume it in supplement form.

Once again, the reason healthy fats are so beneficial is because they promote improved cardiovascular health, reduced inflammation, decreased fat storage, and increased fat metabolism. Personally, I take a handful of almonds everyday to get my monounsaturated fats, take 4 g of omega-3 fatty acid capsules per day for my polyunsaturated source, as well as eating salmon or tuna three times per week. Finally, I add 3 grams of CLA per day, and also try to eat lean red meat or whole eggs 2-3 times per week. Once again, lean red meat and egg yolks are sources of saturated fat, and although deemed unhealthy, are needed periodically to build muscle and sustain adequate hormone production. This nutrition plan ensures I am getting enough healthy fats into my diet.

Summary

- Healthy fats are essential to aid in cardiovascular health, reducing inflammation, and even fat loss.

- If the body does not have adequate fat in its diet, you will actually lose muscle and have a difficult time losing fat.

- Your diet should contain 10-20% of it calories from "healthy fats" which include monounsaturated and polyunsaturated sources. While saturated is deemed unhealthy, moderate consumption 2-3 times per week will ensure adequate hormone production.

- Monounsaturated fats are found in almonds, peanuts and sesame seeds to name a few.

- Polyunsaturated fats include the essential fatty acids. These include the three omega-3 fatty acids (EPA/DHA/alpha-linolenic acids) and omega-6 fatty acids (linoleic acids.) Omega-3, specifically EPA/DHA, is superior, and should be your main focus.

- Conjugated Linoleic Acid (CLA) is an isomer of linoleic acids (Omega-6) and in actuality is a "good" trans-fat. It aids in fat loss by slowing or inhibiting fat storage after meals. Taking 3 grams per day in supplement form is ideal.

- Omega-3 fats can be found in coldwater fish such as salmon and tuna, as well as walnuts, flax seed oil, and in supplement form. The highest concentration of EPA/DHA is found in coldwater fish or fish oil supplements.

- One of the reasons omega-3 fatty acids are so beneficial is because they are metabolized into eicosapentaenoic acid (EPA) and docosahexaenoic acid (DHA).

- Chose the omega-3 fatty acid source that provides the highest yield of EPA/DHA.

- While both are classified as omega-3, the yield of EPA/DHA obtained through cold water fish and fish oil supplements is far superior to that from walnuts and flax seed oil, as they must convert ALA to EPA and DHA. Some individuals can't complete this conversion. Fish and fish oil already have a high concentration of these specific omega-3 fatty acids, which makes them a better choice.

- Rarely combine fat and carbohydrates. Both are energy sources, and can lead to fat accumulation when consumed together.
- Try to avoid fat post workout as it delays absorption of the nutrients you take in.
- I prefer to take a total of 4 g of omega-3 fatty acid capsules and 3 g of CLA spaced throughout the day. In addition, I consume a handful of almonds each day with lean red meat, whole eggs, and salmon a few times each week.
- Understanding fat and how it can aid in your physical transformation is key to achieving your goals.

Fat Sources

1. Salmon (Polyunsaturated)

2. Walnuts (Polyunsaturated)

3. Flax Seed Oil (Polyunsaturated)

4. Peanut Butter (Monounsaturated)

5. Almonds (Monounsaturated)

6. Olive Oil (Monounsaturated)

7. Lean beef steak (Saturated)

8. Venison (Saturated)

9. Whole Eggs (Think of as saturated but also contains cholesterol, mono and poly fats)

Just Remember Each Macronutrient has a purpose:

- **Protein: Growth and Repair**

- **Carbohydrates: Energy**

- **Fat: Energy and Hormone Production**

It's that simple!

Chapter 4

Supplements are just that. They supplement what should already be a solid nutrition and training regimen. Unfortunately, by taking supplements, many believe that they can get away with poor nutritional habits and mediocre training. I will say that I have tried many of the supplements out there, and never once did they make up for poor training or eating habits. If you look around most gyms, those who *really* stand out are the ones who train hard and eat right. Don't get me wrong, I think using supplements judiciously and wisely are very beneficial, but which ones? Below, I will describe what I feel to be the best supplements you should add to your nutrition and training program. Most of the supplement industry is not FDA approved and therefore it is easy to take products that are worthless or can actually harm you. I assure you, I take my health very seriously and feel these supplements are safe and have caused me no harm. **However**, before starting any supplement or training program check with your physician to make sure there are no health factors present that might put you at risk.

The Big 5

1. **Whey Protein:** This can be bought anywhere and we described the various types in the last section on protein. Whey protein is simply a powder sold in various flavors that will make eating healthy that much easier. One scoop usually represents about 120 calories and 25g of protein, with not enough carbohydrates or fat to worry about. The absolute best time to take whey is **immediately** after lifting secondary to its fast-absorption characteristics.

Amount: It is recommended as an athlete to take 1g of protein, per pound of bodyweight, per day. The best times are when you need the quickest absorption, such as breakfast and post workout. I feel it is best to not consume more than half of your daily protein from whey. The other half should consist of animal sources such as eggs, chicken, steak, fish, and turkey. The whey I prefer is Optimum and EAS brands.

2.   Branch Chain Amino Acids (BCAA): Along with glutamine, the BCAA are the most important among the twenty amino acids. This is because they are first to initiate muscle repair and growth, as well as prevent muscle breakdown. The **BCAA's are made up of leucine, valine, and isoleucine.** Leucine is the most vital amino acid in regards to resistance training, as it is the first to initiate repair and protein synthesis after lifting. The BCAA are also the first to be released upon muscle breakdown, to provide the body with fuel in the absence of glucose, as well as to synthesize glutamine that is depleted during exercise. We will talk more about the relationship between BCAA and glutamine in the next section, but for now, lets discuss how branch chain amino acids are broken down to produce fuel.

How BCAA Act As a Fuel Source

Once glucagon is released, a derivative of glycogen and a by-product of BCAA breakdown, called nitrogen, can be combined and shunted to the liver in the form of alanine. This occurs when the body is low on glucose and needs fuel. Here, alanine can be converted into glucose through gluconeogenesis, transported back into the blood, and then used by the body for energy. While BCAA are extracted from muscle tissue to produce fuel, studies have shown that BCAA levels stay stable in the muscle even after this occurs!

What, I thought you said that BCAA are broken down and depleted with exercise? Well they are, but they are quickly re-synthesized in the liver and the process starts all over. **The key point is that muscle is broken down so BCAA can be made available to keep the body running.** Even if the body re-synthesizes more BCAA, *we have already broken down the muscle* *we have worked so hard to build.* So, by supplementing with BCAA, muscle doesn't have to be broken-down as there will be plenty in the bloodstream to be used for fuel and other processes.

Once again, of the three BCAA, leucine is the one most responsible for muscle growth. As we just learned though, it can also be used to produce energy if muscle is broken down. What do you think the bodies first priority is? Energy! If there is a need for energy in the body, then leucine <u>will not</u> be used to build muscle. Rather, it will be used to produce glucose and keep the brain humming along, as glucose is the brains favorite fuel source. So, we need to make sure we have adequate BCAA in our system so the body won't tap into muscle stores.

mTOR

I will take it a step further and talk briefly about **mTOR.** This stands for the **Mammalian Target of Rapamycin,** one of the body's protein synthesis regulators. It is vital for muscle growth and just recently has been given a great deal of attention. mTOR is essentially activated in the presence of high **ATP (adenosine-tri-phosphate)**, one of the bodies immediate energy sources, or when high levels of amino acids are available. It primarily responds to high levels of leucine, which is no surprise as leucine is the BCAA most responsible for muscle growth. While mTOR can be activated independently, with either high energy levels or amino acid availability, the *greatest activation occurs when both are elevated.* **So if ATP levels are high, and the body has adequate amino acids present, then mTOR will have its greatest effect, and the stimulus for muscle growth will be at its maximum.** As you can see, there are numerous things that must happen to initiate muscle growth. Told you it was tough!
One more time…in ENGLISH…...what is needed for muscle growth?

1. There must be **more** protein available than that which is used to keep the body running.

2. BCAA's, specifically leucine, must be present in the blood to inhibit muscle breakdown and initiate repair. If they are present in the blood, then the body won't need to extract them from the muscles and can focus on muscle growth.

3.   The body must have **adequate energy stores in the form of ATP.**

In summary, **we must have plenty of stored energy and amino acids to play with.** If these criteria are met, then mTOR will be stimulated to maximize muscle growth. Of course, you need proper training but we are getting to that!

The "Cravings" Hormone

Leucine has another affect on mTOR in its ability to stimulate the secretion of **leptin.** When mTOR is stimulated by an abundance of leucine, it also activates the release of the hormone leptin from fat cells. **Leptin is a very complicated hormone that essentially controls our appetite, bodyweight, and metabolism.** This hormone is secreted by the fat cells and is responsible for telling us how "full" or "hungry" we are. When we have an adequate amount of body fat, leptin secretion is increased. On the other hand, when we are starving or dieting, the release is dramatically reduced. Anytime we try to lose body fat, the fat cells or adipocytes will release less and less leptin, which severely increases our cravings.

This has been the downfall of many dieters as the urges become to great on prolonged low calorie diets. In fact, over weight individuals have been found to genetically have a down regulation of leptin receptors, and thus have trouble controlling their appetite. The leptin can never lock on to their receptors, and thus, never signals the body that they should be full, no matter how much leptin is released. That's where leucine comes in, as it can induce the feeling of a "fed" state through mTOR activation and secondary leptin release. In essence, consume leucine, and you will feel more full and be less likely to go on binges. This occurs without extra calories or insulin spikes. Thus, fat loss continues, muscle synthesis is enhanced, and we do not plateau.

Summary

- If needed by the body, BCAA will be broken down to synthesize glucose for energy or glutamine for immunity. This is its first priority, and will occur before it considers building muscle. So make sure you always have enough present in your bloodstream.
- Following the proper training protocols, muscle synthesis will occur if all of the bodies basic needs have been met, and excess protein is available.
- If adequate energy reserves are present in the form of ATP, and amino acids are plentiful, specifically leucine, then mTOR can be activated to maximize muscle growth.
- LEUCINE+ ATP + mTOR=maximum muscle gains
- An abundance of leucine can activate mTOR and induce the feeling of a "fed-state," by increasing the secretion of the hormone leptin by fat cells. Leptin release is decreased anytime we start losing body fat and reducing calories, which can often cause us to eat excessively. By consuming leucine and activating mTOR, we can initiate leptin release without consuming more calories.

The Critical Importance of BCAA

We discussed the importance of performing cardio on an empty stomach to maximize fat burning. We also discussed how cortisol can be released in times of stress, such as working out, and when insulin is not present. Should that occur, muscles breaks down to provide fuel, and that is the last thing we want. So how do we get around that? We don't want to spike insulin because that will inhibit our fat burning. We also don't want to consume nothing, as that will increase cortisol and initiate muscle breakdown. The answer lies in BCAA supplementation.

By consuming BCAA before, during, and after your workouts, whether cardio or weights, you will provide an abundance of amino acids to the bloodstream. These can then be used to produce fuel, as well as many other necessary functions, so the body won't have to break down muscle to obtain them. Not only that, it begins the repair process before you are even done working out! Although most quality whey protein supplements contain BCAA, they will not have the same effect as taking them on an empty stomach. That is why I encourage taking BCAA, glutamine, and creatine, all on an empty stomach, 15-30 minutes before a meal. BCAA are definitely a supplement you can't do without.

Amount: I believe you should take a *minimum* of 5-10g of BCAA before and after either cardio or weight training. This will ensure that you do not break muscle down for fuel, as well as getting a head start on tissue repair. If you can afford to do so, consume another 5-10 g during your weight training session. Powdered BCAA tastes horrible, so I strongly urge you to buy one of the combination products on the market. They taste awesome and have grape, watermelon and other flavors, not to mention having other vital supplements such as glutamine added to the mix. The products I have found to be the best tasting and easiest to mix are ICE by Xtreme Formulations and Xtend by Scivation. These both have adequate BCAA and glutamine in their mixes.

3. **Glutamine:** If there is one supplement that shares the importance of BCAA, then its glutamine. While BCAA are most important for muscle repair and protection, this amino acid takes precedence in regards to our immunity. It doesn't stop there, as glutamine also aids in muscle repair and growth, as well as energy production through gluconeogenesis. Glutamine is also the most prolific amino acid in our muscles, as it comprises 60% of a muscles amino acid content. It has also been touted as being able to increase the production of growth hormone, but other studies have shown the effect to be small a best. The primary reason I believe it to be one of the finest supplements, is its ability to increase immunity and aid in muscle repair.

Where It All Started

Glutamine first seemed to gain a good deal of attention when it's benefits were seen in patients suffering from severe burns. The reason it is so beneficial and aided so many burn patients has to do with its property as a major fuel source for immune cells. While studies have shown that the percentage of orally consumed glutamine is found to be small in the blood after consumption, it is only because the digestive cells of the stomach and intestine consume most of it.

I know what you're thinking, "Why then would I want to waste my money if my muscles aren't going to be getting it?" The reason is that *the consumption by these intestinal cells will occur whether we supplement with glutamine or not!* These cells need glutamine to fuel our immune system and keep us healthy. If we don't take in extra glutamine, the body will make sure to break down muscle to provide adequate amounts of glutamine for these cells. That's right, even those of us who don't workout still need glutamine, and the body makes sure it gets it, by breaking down muscle. It does so by pulling available glutamine stores out of the muscle tissue as well as breaking down BCAA to produce more glutamine.

We all know how important BCAA are to muscle growth, so we need to make sure glutamine concentrations are adequate to prevent muscle loss. If we are constantly breaking down muscle, there is no way we will get stronger, stay healthy, or build more muscle.

Glutamine is also a protein synthesis regulator, meaning if it isn't found in adequate concentrations in the muscles, the body will have a hard time building more muscle. So the bottom line is-**supplement with glutamine!** This will ensure that the stomach cells have what they require to increase immunity, muscle concentrations are adequate to stimulate growth, and that BCAA are not broken down to produce more glutamine. More and more studies continue to show that this amino acid is vital for any hard training athlete. In my opinion, it is a necessity.

Amount: I like to take a *minimum* of 5-10g before and after my lifting or cardio workouts. On off days I take 5-10g in the morning. I prefer to get my glutamine from Xtend or ICE as described in the BCAA section, but also like the EAS glutamine product.

4. **Creatine:** Since it came on the market in 1993, no other supplement has been more widely used by athletes. While the vast majority of published studies pertaining to the effects of creatine are positive, it is not a miracle supplement. It is an extremely effective one though, and one that can accelerate your progress dramatically. While lifting weights or exercising, the body uses an immediate form of energy called **adenosine tri-phosphate (ATP)**. We have talked quite a bit about glucose and fat as major energy sources, but remember they are merely "ingredients" to the actual synthesis of ATP. While it isn't important to understand the cycles leading to ATP production, **it is critical to understand that carbohydrates, fats and proteins all eventually lead to ATP production in different ways.** Therefore, anything that can provide more ATP (ie energy) will do nothing but improve our workouts.

That's where creatine comes in. The more creatine you have in your muscles, the faster and more explosive your initial energy can be when running or lifting. That is why so many athletes such as sprinters and football players find it so advantageous.

Now, what many people don't realize is that the by-products of amino acids form creatine. What that essentially means is, **we produce it naturally.** In fact, most people synthesize about a gram a day, and those who eat red meat synthesize even more. 95% of the creatine in our body is stored in skeletal muscle, with the other 5% in the liver, kidneys, brain and testes. When energy is needed, ATP will cleave off one of it's phosphate groups, becoming ADP, and thus provide the body with immediate energy. Creatine phosphate, with the donation of its phosphate group, allows the adenosine-*di*-phosphate to become adenosine-*tri*-phosphate again, much quicker than more ATP can be produced from glucose and fat metabolism. Thus, you recover quicker secondary to the quick re-synthesis of ATP (Fig 8).

Fig. 8

Lift Weight→ATP used→ADP +P is left over→

→*Creatine donates phosphate to ADP→ATP produced

again

Creatine has also been directly related to enhanced exercise performance. The more creatine in a given muscle, the better it will be able to complete a given task. Also, fast twitch muscle fibers, the ones that are most responsible for growth and strength, contain the highest concentration of creatine. Coincidence? I think not when we look at the benefits it yields to football players, track stars, and other explosive athletes.

To Load or Not To Load

One of the major question marks in the supplementation of creatine is whether to load or not. The loading theory refers to taking 20g a day for 5 days and then following that with a maintenance dose of 5g per day. Recent research has shown that after 48 hrs, subjects were excreting the majority of their creatine intake. So, it is of the mindset now to just take 5-10g a day, preferably pre and post workout, with no loading dose. In doing this, the body will not convert nearly as much creatine to its immediate metabolite creatinine, which is excreted by the body. Now, here's the cool part. Once creatine is loaded into the muscles, it will stay loaded, for up to one month, without further creatine intake! So, if you want to cycle creatine, take it for 3 months and then stop for 4-5 weeks. There will still be some creatine present in your muscles for the month you take off.

Important note: Creatine has been shown to cause dehydration in some and therefore one should make sure they are properly hydrated while taking this supplement.

Amount: I like to take 5-10g before and after my workout. On off days I take 5-10g in the morning. I prefer AST or EAS creatine.

5. **Omega-3-fatty acids:** These are the types of **essential** good fats we talked about earlier. They are called **essential fatty acids** simply because your body cannot produce them alone, and therefore must obtain them from food sources. It has been said that you can obtain all the omega 3 fatty acids you need by consuming cold water fish, such as tuna or salmon 2-3 times per week. However, in the world we live in, it can be difficult to find the time to cook these cold-water fish. So, by taking 3-4g per day of omega-3-fatty acids or "fish oil" capsules, you will get the essential fatty acids that you need. These will improve the function and lubrication of your joints, increase testosterone, support the use of body fat as fuel, and greatly decrease your risk of cardiovascular disease. For a more thorough discussion on these essential fatty acids, go back and review the section on fats. I consider them one of the most important supplements.

Amount: Take a total of 3-4 g per day of fish oil capsules with meals. Doing this everyday is the equivalent of eating salmon or tuna 2-3 times per week. Nature Made is the company I use most often in regards to my fish oil capsules.

Other Worthwhile Supplements

<u>Vitargo:</u>
By now I am sure you realize simple carbohydrates should be avoided at all times except those surrounding the workout period, and in some cases breakfast. Simple carbohydrates are most important, no matter the goal, during the post workout period. The ensuing insulin spike is essential to shuttle nutrients into muscles and cells to initiate the repair process. There is one problem some trainees face though in regards to consuming a high amount of simple carbohydrates post workout. That is stomach discomfort. Many post workout formulations include a high amount of these "simple sugars" in their formulas, with creatine often added. There is an incredible formula however that not only increases the absorption of nutrients, but also does so with out sugar! This magic formula is called vitargo.

Vitargo is a patented, high molecular weight carbohydrate made from Swedish waxy maize starch. It essentially is a complex carbohydrate. I know what you are thinking, "You said complex carbohydrates were not ideal post workout!" I stand by that, but in this case, it is an exception. The reason being is that it is a high molecular weight carbohydrate with low osmolality. When you consume dextrose (a.k.a glucose) in many post workout drinks, the molecular weight is much smaller than vitargo. So, before dextrose leaves the stomach on its way to the small intestine, it will pull water back into the stomach. This is why so many trainees suffer from bloating and cramps after consuming their "high sugar" post workout drink.

Yet another reason consuming dextrose is not as beneficial as vitargo is the rate at which it gets to the bloodstream. Although it is true that it will get there sooner than "normal" complex carbohydrates, it won't do it as fast as vitargo. In addition, if you consume creatine in your post workout shake, the dextrose will hit the bloodstream before creatine, and thus cause the majority of the insulin spike without creatine or other supplements even being present! If that happens, you will waste some of the creatine you have added to your shake. This is why I consume my creatine, glutamine, and BCAA on an empty stomach, at least 15 minutes before my post-workout meal. When you consume vitargo, the molecular weight is so high that it acts as a pump, and pulls creatine into the small intestine with it, much faster than consuming conventional glucose.

How Does This Work?

The reason vitargo works as such is due to its high molecular weight and low osmolality. The lower the osmolality, the faster it gets through the stomach and into the bloodstream. These characteristics make it a superior post-workout carbohydrate source. Don't get me wrong; you can still achieve tremendous gains from Gatorade or dextrose in your post workout drink. In fact, I use that combination most of the time, as I usually don't suffer any stomach discomfort. Our goal is simply to ensure an adequate insulin spike the most efficient way we can and give you options. I have found that I feel more fullness in my muscles and more energy when using a waxy maize source, but both can be effective. Try it, you may experience gains like never before!

Amount: Usually 2 scoops in 20 oz of water post workout. Ideal use is after weight training to replenish glycogen and nutrients in the muscles. Vitargo CGL my Nutrex is my favorite product.

Multivitamin: These are vital. Why? Because you will be training at a level far above the average person. Thus, you need to supply your body with enough of the vitamins and minerals it needs to keep your immunity up, as well as build muscle and lose fat. If your sick, the body will use its energy to cure the illness before it decides to improve your physique. I recommend a good multi-vitamin that has 100%DV for each of its respective vitamins. There are many out there, so find a good quality one that works for you.

Amount: One quality multivitamin per day by Nature Made is what I use.

Glucosamine/Chondroitin: I have become a firm believer in these of late. They have been shown to prevent loss of cartilage and even aid the body in rebuilding it. Tendons and ligaments are poorly vascularized. Therefore if you injure one or start to degenerate, you can understand why it takes so long to recover. Blood brings factors that aid in repair, and with limited blood supply, the process is slow. By taking a good glucosamine/chondrotin supplement, you can decrease the risk of degeneration and thus prevent injury. While not FDA approved or a miracle supplement, these definitely seem to make my joints feel better.

Amount: Some supplements provide the required dose in 1-2 tablets and others require 3 servings per day. The bottom line is to get 1500 mg of Glucosamine and 1200 mg Chondroitin per day. Nature Made makes a very good product and one should be careful to choose reputable companies as some falsify the amount of product placed in each bottle.

Vitamin C and E: I firmly believe in taking 500mg of vitamin C and 400 I.U. of vitamin E in the morning and at night. These two vitamins are essential to aid in your immunity. We will be in a stressful state, and need all the help we can get to combat colds and other "bugs." Although many might think this is overkill, the top trainers I have worked with all had one thing in common: they all believed in supplementing with vitamin C and vitamin E. Take them, they do help!

Amount: I take 400 IU of vitamin E and 500mg of vitamin C twice per day. I do cardiovascular and resistance training in the same day, and feel that I need more insurance to protect my health. At a bare minimum, I believe you should consume these vitamins at least once per day to ensure adequate immunity and overall health. Again, Nature Made is my company of choice.

There you have it, the basics to supplementation. Although there are hundred's of products on the market, these have stood the test of time. They are basic, and yet the most effective products you can add to your training. Combining a solid workout program, with consistent nutrition and supplementation, is the key to taking your physique to the next level.

Supplements for Fat Loss

This topic might catch the eye of many of you as we are all looking for that little extra kick to aid in fat loss. Let me make one think clear to start with; ***nothing is as important as training and diet***. I think many individuals hear about the latest and greatest diet pill and think all their problems are solved. However, without consuming the proper nutrients and having an effective workout program, these products ultimately fail. Worse, the person who bought the product assumes if "this" didn't work, then it just isn't possible for them to lose weight. Wrong! Nutrition is at the forefront to getting lean, followed by training and finally supplementation. In saying that, there are many supplements that can accelerate your fat loss. Instead of going out and buying any number of the fat loss products out there, lets first understand them.

Understanding Fat Loss Supplements

The loss of fat is regulated by **adrenoreceptors**, which are essentially binding sites for specific hormones called **catecholamines**. Catecholamines are a subject that we didn't discuss in the section on hormones, as I felt it would make more sense to describe them here. They, along with GH, are the most important "fat burners" that we naturally produce. Catecholamines in fact inhibit the release of insulin, which as you know is essential to increase fat loss. We have all heard of the sympathetic and parasympathetic nervous system. The "fight or flight" response is triggered by an activation of the sympathetic nervous system by these same catecholamines. It is what excites us or gets us going. **Adrenaline and noradrenaline, otherwise known as epinephrine (E) and norepinephrine (NE), are what specifically make up the catecholamines.** They are produced by the adrenal glands, which anatomically sit above the kidneys. As you'll soon see, the release of these chemicals by the body is a major catalyst to initiate the loss of body fat.

How Do Catecholamines Initiate Fat Loss?

To initiate fat loss, catecholamines must first bind to an adrenoreceptor on the surface of a fat cell, in a lock and key type of relationship. Now, we must realize that not all adrenoreceptors are created equal. There are *two alpha and three beta adrenoreceptors*. When catecholamines bind beta or alpha-1 receptors, fatty acids are released, and are eventually used as energy in various organs. More simply stated, we burn fat! When catecholamines bind alpha-2 receptors, fat loss is actually inhibited.

They Can't Do It Alone

Now, they can't do it alone though and actually need the help of HSL to "split" the fatty acids from glycerol, and release them into the bloodstream. Therefore, the binding of catecholamines to beta-adrenergic receptors is another way to stimulate the secretion of glucagon and HSL (hormone sensitive lipase). HSL is always the "middle man," with the end result being the use of fat for fuel.

Other Adrenoreceptors

There are also alpha-receptors, specifically alpha-1 and alpha-2. Compared to alpha-2, alpha-1 is the receptor most responsible for fat loss when bound, albeit at a much-reduced rate compared to beta-receptors. *Now, here's the catch and an important one.* **While beta-receptors and alpha-1 can initiate fat loss, alpha-2, when bound, actually inhibits it!** So we must inhibit the catecholamines from attaching to alpha-2 adrenoreceptors if we want to continue burning fat. These alpha-2 receptors are very prominent in the upper thighs, "love-handle" region, and stomach. Essentially, the areas we have the most difficulty toning up. It has in fact been shown that catecholamine action in adipose tissue is greatly reduced in obese individuals. Reasons this might occur are the increased expression of alpha-2 receptors (which promote fat storage), decreased expression of beta-receptors (which stimulate fat utilization), and decreased expression of HSL.

In Summary:

Stimulation of beta-receptors and alpha-1 can be thought of as the "on" switch for fat loss, while stimulation of alpha-2 receptors can be considered the "off" switch.

Once catecholamines bind to adrenoreceptors, HSL is the final ingredient to ensuring fat is used as energy. In fact as we age, and in some obese individuals, the levels of HSL are far below the norm and therefore, fat loss is greatly reduced. We need all the pieces of the fat burning puzzle to be present if we want to maximize our success. The key then is to ensure the natural production of catecholamines (epinephrine/nor epinephrine), which leads to increased HSL activity and fat loss.

Why Is It So Hard to Lose Fat?

Many have trouble losing weight if they are obese and become frustrated very quickly. If we can understand "why" though, it will make the task much easier. Obesity can cause "epinephrine-resistance" much like a diabetic can suffer from insulin resistance. Some diabetics suffer from increased blood sugar because the receptors for insulin have been destroyed, or are non responsive to insulin. Thus, insulin can't bind and cause an uptake of glucose into the body for its basic needs. The same goes for epinephrine in obese patients. Increased insulin causes destruction of beta- receptors and a severe reduction in HSL, which remember aids in fat loss. So, if there are non-functioning beta-receptors, which must be bound by catecholamines to initiate fat loss, no amount of NE or HSL will matter. Who cares if you have a key if there is no lock? The secret then is to slowly wake these beta-receptors up, with lower blood sugars and exercise. This will increase catecholamine and HSL activity, inhibit insulin release, and accelerate fat loss.

This is why the now banned drug ephedra was so successful in aiding thousands to lose body fat. It directly increased the amount of catecholamines produced by the body, which as you now know increases fat loss. Now, just because we understand how the body burns fat, doesn't mean it will be easy. Fat can be hard to burn and the body just doesn't want to give up fat unless it has too. So, we are going to have to make it. How? Well, we have talked a bit about this already but if you add a "fat burner", which will increase the amount of catecholamines, along with ingredients we'll talk about next, then you have a potent combination. You will, notice I say will…be ripped!

"Fat Burning" Ingredients

Nearly all-fat burners on the market now contain ingredients that will increase your production of catecholamines. As far as supplements go, **synephrine** is a substitute many companies use to initiate catecholamine release. Synephrine directly stimulates the beta-3 receptor, while not affecting beta-1 or beta-2. This reduces any heart problems that may occur with indirect acting beta-agonists such as ephedra. Indirect acting drugs such as ephedra hit all the receptors, so while fat loss is still occurring, other side effects may put your health in jeopardy. This is one of the main reasons it was taken off the market. While synephrine is safer than ephedra or other indirect acting agents, **everyone should check with his or her medical doctor before starting any weight loss supplement.** Things such as hypertension and cardiovascular disease could potentially become worse on supplements that increase sympathetic activity, despite being great fat loss tools. Be smart, and check with your doctor first.

Anything Else?

What else should a quality fat burner contain? Well, one of the best supplements to accelerate fat loss is **caffeine**. It is in fact the number one drug in America. Drug? That's right, it is addicting. But, it increases awareness, energy, and also "sweet talks" the body into giving up some fat for energy. Another supplement, **Gugglsterones**, are made from a plant native to India, and increase fat loss by stimulating the thyroid hormones. Essentially, they raise your core body temperature, and therefore your metabolic rate. Many fat loss supplements have them included in small doses and some not at all.

Yohimbine is an alpha-2 receptor blocker, or antagonist, and thus inhibits fat deposition in your lower body and love handle region. Again, these are the locations where the concentration of alpha-2 receptors is highest. Remember that NE, a catecholamine, binds to both alpha *and* beta-receptors. Binding to alpha-2 however is not a good thing in regards to fat loss. Essentially, once NE binds to alpha 2 receptors, the body stops producing NE. It acts as its own negative feedback loop, essentially shutting itself down. There are large numbers of alpha-2 receptors in the hips, butt, thighs, and in the stomach region, namely the areas we most want to tone up. The task of burning fat is made easier then when we inhibit the binding of catecholamines to alpha-2 receptors with yohimbine.

A final supplement, which can aid in fat loss, is **green tea**. Green tea is rich in catechins, specifically epigallocatechin gallate (EGCG), which is thought to inhibit an enzyme that breaks down NE. Therefore, if green tea can prevent NE from being broken down, there will be more of it present to catalyze fat burning. Green tea also contains caffeine, which as you know, can also aid in reducing our levels of body fat.

In summary, synephrine and similar compounds increase the release of NE, caffeine increases energy and the use of fat for fuel, gugglsterons increase thyroid function which raises metabolism, yohimbine is an alpha-2 blocker which prevents binding of catecholamines to alpha-2 receptors, and green tea contains epigallocatechin gallate (EGCG) which inhibits the breakdown of NE. Once again, there is no substitute for diet and exercise, but adding synephrine, caffeine, gugglsterones, yohimbine, and green tea can greatly increase your fat loss results.

Be Careful

If anyone has high blood pressure or poor health, I advise staying away from these natural aids for fat loss. You can accomplish a great deal with sound diet and exercise, and in no way are these products a substitute. No supplement is more abused than fat burners, as many take them and continue to eat poorly. In this case you do nothing but blunt your receptors, so that when you do get on the wagon and decide to eat clean, you will notice they aren't helping at all. Only take them after checking with your physician, if you are on a specific program to get lean, and never for more than 12 weeks. Once again, they accelerate fat loss, but should be used accordingly.

IS THERE ANOTHER WAY?

I believe that if one is serious about fat loss, but doesn't want to take the above ingredients found in most fat burners, then there is another way. There is an amino acid-like supplement called **acetly-l-carnitine (ALC).** Many in fact use ALC in conjunction with the supplements mentioned above. It has been shown to increase everything from sex drive to burning fat. We must remember that before the fat burning process can begin, the fat cells must release fatty acids into the bloodstream. From there, they must be transported to the mitochondria of the cell to be used as energy. This is when we actually begin to lose fat. So, what does that have to do with ALC?

Everything actually! ALC accelerates the passage of these fatty acids into the mitochondria, and thus increases fat loss. HSL is needed to initiate the release of fatty acids, and then **ALC accelerates the transport to the cells mitochondria.** Personally, when trying to get leaner, I take 1g before weight training and 1g before cardio. I also take caffeine every morning in the form of a diet Pepsi or green tea. Coffee is even better, and no-dose works great. If you add a fat burner to this combination, hold off on the caffeine as most fat burners have around 200mg in them. A great starting combination is caffeine and ALC. Then as you transform your body, you can make changes along the way, as you now know the secrets to fat loss supplementation.

Fig 9. Fat Loss Flow Chart

Catecholamine (NE/E) release→Bind to

Adrenoreceptors→Glucagon and HSL is released→Fatty acids

are released to blood→ ALC transports fatty acids to cell's

mitochondria→Fat is burned!!!!!!!!!!!!!!!!!!!!!!!

Summary of General Supplements:

Whey Protein: initiates repair and protects muscles from breakdown.
BCAA: initiates repair and protects muscles from breakdown.
Glutamine: aids in immunity, muscle repair, growth, and protection.
Creatine: immediate energy source.
Omega-3-fatty acids: cardiovascular health, joint health, fat loss, and
  hormone production.
Vitargo: made from waxy maize starch and used as a post workout
  carbohydrate source.
Multivitamin: overall health.
Glucosamine/Chondroitin: joint repair and protection.
Vitamin C and Vitamin E: immunity/overall health.

Summary of Fat Loss Supplements:

Catecholamines (NE/E): when released bind adrenoreceptors which
  are either alpha or beta.
• Binding of catecholamines to alpha-1 or any beta-receptors
  initiates fat loss.
• Binding of catecholamines to alpha-2 inhibits fat loss.
Caffeine: increases energy and the use of fat for fuel.
Gugglsterones: increase thyroid function, which raises metabolism to
  burn more fat.

Yohimbine: is an alpha-2 blocker, which prevents NE form binding to alpha-2 sites. This increases fat metabolism.

Green Tea: contains epigallocatechin gallate (EGCG), which has been shown to aid in fat loss by inhibiting the breakdown of NE.

Hormone Sensitive Lipase (HSL): aids in freeing fatty acids from their glycerol backbone and into the bloodstream.

Acetyl-l-carnitine (ALC): aids in the transport of fatty acids from the bloodstream to the mitochondria of various cells so they can be used for energy.

Chapter 5

CREATING THE IDEAL NUTRITION AND SUPPLEMENT PROGRAM

Now that we have covered the macronutrients and general supplements, what next? Training right? Well, not so fast. We will get there but for now, we need to set up a nutrition program to allow for the most significant gains. Remember, what we look like is 75% nutrition. We must realize that our nutrition program will change depending on our goals. If getting lean while slowly building muscle is our main focus, then I favor what I call a "carbohydrate cycle," which we will cover at the end of this chapter. If gaining muscle mass and strength is our primary goal, I believe it calls for a different protocol. The training, I am sorry to say, is not that complicated, as long as you follow the principles I'll outline later in this book. Our training is merely the stimulus, supplements help push us along, but nutrition is where its at. Lets start with nutrient timing, then figure out exactly how many calories, carbohydrates, proteins, and fats we need to get started.

The Anabolic Window

We have outlined many of the keys to making tremendous gains and changes in our physique. The area I want to go into more detail now, deals with the time frame I call the **anabolic window.** There is absolutely no time when nutrition is more important than the hours surrounding your workout. The anabolic window consists of the 1-hour preceding your workout, the workout period itself, and finally, the 1-hour window after you train. Many think that working out by itself will build a solid, healthy physique, but nothing could be further from the truth. In fact, if you train hard and don't eat correctly, you will actually do more damage than if you didn't train at all!

The reason behind the last statement is simple. Resistance training causes damage to the bodies muscle tissue. This in itself is the only way you can get stronger, leaner, or bigger. The muscle must be broken down or damaged through stressors (lifting) and then rebuilt with proper nutrition. If you lift hard, and don't take in adequate nutrients to initiate the repair process, you will actually make the damaged tissue weaker.

Think of wanting to take your current home and reconstructing it, to make it the home of your dreams. You tear it down all day Saturday, but then are left with nothing but bricks, boards, and debris all over the place. You then realize you have no clue how to build it back to its current state, much less make it better. The same goes for your physical transformation. If you only know how to train hard, but have no idea how to reconstruct your physique, why train in the first place?

I know we have talked about the importance of protein, carbohydrates, and fats, but using those in the right proportions during the anabolic window is vital to your success. I firmly believe that the reason many athletes don't change more consistently, and for the better, is because they fail to maximize a time frame that the body is most conducive to the absorption of nutrients.

Once again, the thing to remember is there is not a more important time for optimal nutrition than the hours surrounding a workout (sick of me saying that yet?). Training with weights is hard on the body, and as we know, stress hormones, such as cortisol, are released anytime the body perceives a stressful state. When cortisol is present, muscle breaks down, fat is held onto, and positive changes stop. However, **by taking in nutrients in the 3-hour window surrounding your weight training, the results will amaze you!** In the past, I for one would have great success burning fat in the morning on an empty stomach, but would always feel flat while lifting. Then I started this nutrient system and was amazed. I had better pumps, my soreness was dramatically reduced, and I actually could see the changes occurring. Let me explain why.

A Basic Understanding

The instance you initiate trauma to the body, through injury or weight training, cortisol will be released. However, if you consume the nutrients and supplements I will be prescribing, a cascade of positive things begin to happen. Cortisol is inhibited by insulin, released after consuming the high GI carbohydrates, glutamine, and BCAA you will be drinking during your workout. Insulin and amino acids, as you know, oppose cortisol. Insulin also initiates the uptake of valuable nutrients such as protein, BCAA, creatine, and glutamine, while you are lifting! Therefore, they can begin to initiate repair while you train, as well as providing energy to fuel your workout.

At no time during the day will there be more blood flowing through your muscles than during a weight-training workout. So, why not capitalize on that, and place nutrients in the body at a time they are most likely to be used by the muscles? The muscle receptors before, during, and ___**within 60 minutes**___ of the completion of your workout are primed to initiate repair and take in any nutrient they can find. They are literally like sponges. Each minute that passes after training makes the fat cell receptors more sensitive to insulin, and eventually, with enough time, more sensitive that the muscle receptor sites. Remember, insulin can shuttle nutrients into fat cells as well! That's when you have lost your chance to make the most gains, and will be fighting to just hold onto the muscle you have, much less produce more.

While it is true that all you need before cardio is a BCAA/glutamine mix, resistance training is a completely different ball game. This is the time when you shouldn't be concerned with inhibiting fat loss. In fact, you should be more concerned with protecting and building your muscles. Remember, muscle burns fat all day long, the more you have, the more fat you'll burn. A small amount of simple carbohydrates consumed during your workout will not derail your fat burning efforts, and do nothing but improve muscle growth. We are not talking about a large number of carbohydrates, just enough to keep you from becoming catabolic. The nutrients you consume will inhibit muscle loss, and give you a head start to the major repair that will occur in the hours following your workout.

What Should I Take?

Before performing cardio in the morning, I only consume 1g of acetyl-l-carnitine, caffeine, 5-10g BCAA, and 5-10g glutamine. When its time to lift though, **I consume different and specific nutrients surrounding my workout .** I assure you that you will not put on fat with these meals, provided you are working hard. Everything you consume will benefit you.

Here's what I recommend:

1. About 1 hour before you lift, consume 20-40 g of whey protein, 15-25 g of complex carbohydrates, and 5-10 g of healthy fats. Normally I don't combine fats and carbohydrates but in this case, the extra energy and digestion slowing effects of the added fats will help with energy for the workout. I like 20-40 g of whey and 1 slice of Ezekiel bread with a tbsp peanut butter. Fruit is another option.

2. Immediately before you lift, start consuming a large drink mix made with water, 20 g of simple carbohydrates such as a tbsp Gatorade powder, 10-20g of BCAA, 10 g creatine and 10 g of glutamine. Remember that glutamine, creatine, and BCAA are best absorbed on a fairly empty stomach, and your last meal will have been 1 hour before.

3. During your workout, continue sipping this cocktail and just add more water as your bottle gets low.

4. IMMEDIATELY after you lift, consume 40 g of whey protein and 50-60 g of fast digesting carbohydrates such as a 32 oz Gatorade or 2 scoops of Vitargo.

These nutrients when consumed as stated will build muscle fast! They will supply the needed nutrients, in appropriate amounts, when you need them most. It is important to only consume this meal set-up on days you lift. If you train intensely, you will still produce growth hormone, build muscle, and burn fat. If you are trying to lose a large amount of body fat however, or get lean by a specific date, I would eliminate the 20g of simple carbohydrates during your lift. This will ensure that the body taps into fat as quickly as possible. Muscle loss won't be a problem as the BCAA and glutamine you take in will protect your muscles, and the small amount of complex carbohydrates, creatine, and healthy fats consumed will supply you with enough energy to get you through.

Remember, **cutting out simple carbohydrates during your training session should *only* occur when your primary goal is losing fat quickly.** Muscle gains are much more likely when the simple carbohydrates are added to the workout drink mix, but we must cater each program to the individual. In most cases you can consume the workout carbohydrates, and still ensure adequate fat loss by not consuming carbohydrates more than two hours after working out. This holds true, no matter the goal.

Body Fat Loss and the GLUT-4 Receptor

Now that we have been preaching the absolute need for an insulin spike post workout, there may be one exception. We should all be aware at this point as to the difficulty of losing body fat if insulin levels are increased. Those who have body fat loss as their primary goal, *must* keep insulin levels stable throughout the day. The concern of many though is not absorbing nutrients post workout without the insulin spike. It's a catch-22. One of the reasons that many obese individuals have difficulty losing weight is because they have a reduced sensitivity to insulin. The body has gotten so accustomed to high amounts of sugar in the blood, that it takes an excess amount of insulin to even initiate the absorption of nutrients. Essentially, their GLUT-4 muscle receptors have been down regulated.

What Is A GLUT-4?

GLUT-4 receptors are found inside both fat cells and muscle cells. Whenever insulin is released and binds to a cell membrane, GLUT-4 receptors travel to the surface of their respective cells and allow for the uptake of glucose into the cell. **These are the receptors that make it possible for each one of us to absorb nutrients.** If you exercise, or ideally, lift weights, the <u>receptors on muscle cells will become much more sensitive than those on fat cells.</u> If you don't exercise or lift, then the opposite holds true, and fat cells are more likely to absorb glucose. Hence, making you fatter (Fig 10). So, we need to lift to increase the sensitivity of the muscle receptor sites and decrease the likelihood that fat will get its share of the glucose floating around. **This may be one of the most powerful reasons to engage in a resistance-training program, whether you are male or female.**

Fig. 10

1) Don't Lift Weights:

Glut-4 Sensitivity on Fat Cell > Glut-4 sensitivity on Muscle Cell

2) Lift Weights:

Glut-4 sensitivity on Fat Cell < Glut-4 Sensitivity on Muscle Cell

I know what you're thinking, won't we be wasting our time if we can't absorb nutrients post workout? Don't we need insulin? Well, not necessarily, here's the trick. Anytime you lift weights, the muscles will release calcium. This calcium release will trigger the GLUT-4 receptors on muscles to prepare for absorption. Will it be as great as if you consumed a high GI carbohydrate? No. Will it allow you to absorb nutrients AND keep insulin levels low to keep fat burning accelerated? Yes.

In summary, if you are holding onto a lot of body fat and reducing that is your primary goal, then stay away from high GI foods, even post workout. The calcium release following weight training will initiate the absorption of nutrients, which starts the repair process. Post-workout, consume a low GI food like oatmeal with your whey protein and add a little splenda for flavor. This makes it seem like you are actually eating sugar, and it will reduce your cravings. It also keeps insulin levels more stable, and will not hinder your fat loss efforts.

As you lean out, you can add more high GI foods and drinks back into your anabolic window, which will really accelerate muscle gains. BCAA, glutamine, and creatine are still required and must be consumed before, during, and after lifting. They will not dramatically affect insulin levels.

We are trying to inhibit a massive insulin spike, not accelerate muscle loss, which is exactly what will happen without BCAA and glutamine.

Nutrition Protocol with Body Fat Loss as Primary Goal:

1. About 1 hour before you lift, consume 20-40 g of whey protein and 15 g of complex carbohydrates. I like 40 g of whey and 1 slice of Ezekiel bread. In those who desire dramatic fat loss, I hold off on the extra fat here.

2. 15 minutes before you lift, start consuming a drink mix made with 20 oz of water, 20g of BCAA, 10 g creatine and 10 g of glutamine. Remember that glutamine, creatine, and BCAA are best absorbed on a fairly empty stomach and your last meal will have been about 1 hour before. Once again, I pulled the 20 g of simple carbohydrates out of the mix to enhance fat burning.

3. During your workout, continue sipping this cocktail and just add more water as your bottle gets low.

4. IMMEDIATELY after you lift, consume 40 g of whey protein and 30-50g of complex carbohydrates, such as oatmeal with splenda.

Determining Caloric Intake and Macronutrient Ratios

If your reading this book, you most likely want to attain a muscular, lean physique. As I stated at the beginning of this book, gaining muscle and losing fat is a process that takes time, determination, and patience. There are no shortcuts. Without proper nutrition though, you don't have a chance.

Determining the amount of calories we should consume can be a tricky endeavor. We now know what to consume in the time surrounding our workout, what about the other meals? Do we eat more protein, more fat, or more carbohydrates? I have found that the **baseline caloric intake an**

individual needs is best found by taking your bodyweight (BW) x 12-15.
Now, whether you focus more on 12 or 15 depends on the goal. If getting
leaner is your primary goal, then focus on the lower end. If gaining more
muscle takes precedent, focus more towards 15. This will give you a baseline
caloric intake to get started. *There is no perfect program, as everybody has
different metabolisms, training programs, and body types.* The only way to see
how many calories you need is too document how many you consume, and
then see how your body changes.

I have found that this system works rather well though. Lets say a trainee
weighs 200 lbs and wants to gain quality muscle mass. Their caloric intake
should start at about 3000 calories per day (200 x15). If a 150 trainee wants
to get leaner, they should start at approximately 1800 calories per day (150
x 12). If getting leaner and losing body fat is your goal, then you **must burn
more than you consume.** To gain lean mass or weight, you must increase
the amount of calories you take in. **Simply consume more than you burn.**
This is why it is good to find out how many calories you need to maintain
your weight based on your activity level and body type. If consuming 2500
calories per day keeps you at a stable weight, you know you will have to
consume less than that to lose weight and more to gain. It's that simple.

A very important piece of advice for those new to training are to keep the
same caloric intake for two weeks to see how you adapt. Only then will
you understand how your body is adapting to the caloric intake you are
consuming. Then you can make changes depending on your ultimate goal.
Many make the mistake of eating a baseline caloric intake forever and never
gain quality weight. The body needs a surplus of calories to push past old
limits and therefore, should be more than your baseline intake. So, if you are
eating 3000 calories and not gaining, then increase the calories. If you are
consuming 2400 and not losing, then drop them or increase your activity
level. Eventually you will figure out how many calories you need to gain
muscle mass or lose appreciable amounts of body fat.

Macronutrient Ratios

Now, when in comes to ratios of macronutrients to consume, I like to
start with the 40/40/20 rule. This means, in regards to your total caloric

intake, that you should consume 40 % protein, 40% carbohydrates, and 20% healthy fats as a starting point. **Remember that carbohydrates and proteins represent 4 calories per gram, and fats represent 9 calories per gram.** This equals approximately 260 g of protein, 260 g of carbohydrates, and 60 g of fat for a trainee consuming 2600 calories per day. These calories should be consumed over 6-8 meals, with the majority of your carbohydrate consumption at breakfast, and surrounding the workout period. This will ensure that they are used for recovery and energy, rather than fat accumulation. In the evenings, you should limit your carbohydrate consumption with the exception of green vegetables, as you can eat as many of these as you want. This will ensure little fat accumulation and plenty of fiber to slow digestion. The only exception would be if you train at night, and need to consume your shakes and meals surrounding the anabolic window.

The types of macronutrients you should consume are as follows.

- Focus on complex carbohydrates at all meals except post-workout.
- Consume mostly fibrous carbohydrates at night (i.e. green vegetables), along with healthy fats and protein.
- Try and consume the majority of your carbohydrates at breakfast, and during the anabolic window.
- It is also important to consume a slow digesting protein, such as casein, along with a healthy fat source immediately before bed. This is to ensure a slow release of amino acids throughout the night, when the body has no nutrient intake. The casein protein and fats will slow digestion, along with the vegetables you should be eating for dinner. Many fail to gain muscle simply because they don't take this nighttime shake, and therefore don't provide the muscles with the tools needed for repair. Cottage cheese or casein whey powder is my favorite protein source at night, secondary to their slow release characteristics.

Remember that you grow and repair while you sleep -more than any other time of day. Doesn't it make sense that you need a quality nutrient source to aid in this recovery? Nighttime casein protein meals, mixed with a tbsp of healthy fat, such as flax seed oil or peanut butter, will ensure you maximize your muscle gains. Also, don't forget your simple carbohydrates post workout. This initiates the repair process and inhibits the stress hormones such as cortisol.

Below is an Example Of A Baseline Nutrition Program I have followed before. Getting leaner while slowly building muscle was my primary objective.

Baseline Meal Plan for a 200-pound male athlete trying to lose body fat AND gain muscle

Meal 1: 30 g complex carbohydrates/40 g protein/10-15 grams simple carbohydrates
Add 5-10 g healthy fats

½ cup oatmeal
Tbsp honey or ½ cup fruit
40 g whey protein
10-12 almonds

Meal 2: 30 g protein/ add 10 g healthy fats
30 g whey protein
Tbsp peanut butter

Meal 3: 40 g protein/30 g complex carbohydrates/ 20 g simple carbohydrates
6 oz chicken
2 slices Ezekiel bread
1 piece of fruit

1 hr Pre-workout: 15-20 g complex carbohydrates/40 g protein/add 5-10 g healthy fats
1 slice Ezekiel bread
40 g whey protein
Tbsp peanut butter

15 minutes pre-workout and sip throughout workout:
20 g BCAA
10 g glutamine
10g creatine
20 g simple carbohydrates (tbsp Gatorade powder)

Meal 4: Post Workout: 60 g simple carbohydrates/40 g protein
32 oz Gatorade or 2 scoops vitargo
40 g whey

Meal 5: 30 g protein/30 g complex carbohydrates/veggies (all you can eat)
4-6 oz steak/chicken/or salmon
½ cup brown rice
Veggies

Meal 6: 30 g casein protein/add 10 g healthy fats
30 g casein protein or 1 cup cottage cheese
Tbsp peanut butter or 10-12 almonds

Totals:
Calories: 2660
260 g protein
225 g carbohydrates
50 g fat

* Eat as many _green_ veggies as you can and desire. Corn and carrots, while healthy, are much more dense in carbohydrates. Vegetables in general will aid in stabilizing insulin levels, keep you full longer, and increase your overall health.

Dr. Eyad H. Yehyawi

Macronutrient Intake for the Obese

Is it possible to consume a low amount of carbohydrates and still gain muscle? Absolutely-provided your protein and healthy fat intake is optimal. This section applies to those who gain weight easily, are 50 pounds overweight, or have body fat over 20%.

In this case, consuming excess protein, moderate amounts of healthy fats, and reducing carbohydrate intake is the key to success. The results will be a significant loss of body fat, increased muscle, and better insulin sensitivity. **I recommend a baseline caloric intake starting at BW x 10-12**, with protein intake around 50%, healthy fats around 30%, and carbohydrates around 20%. The **carbohydrates should be mostly complex, and only consumed at breakfast, pre, and post workout.** Protein should approach 300-350 g per day, and healthy fats 60-100 g. Carbohydrates will be anywhere from 90-120 grams-but no more. The body will eventually learn to use fat as an energy source and that is exactly how you will start getting leaner. Insulin output must be kept low.

Increased protein is needed to ensure muscle is not broken down, as well as to keep you feeling full longer. Healthy fats will keep you energetic and full, as well as keep natural hormone production up. The carbohydrates you do consume, and the times you consume them, are to simply allow energy for your workout, and to inhibit cortisol in the morning when you awake. Again, BCAA and glutamine are absolutely essential.

The following meal plan is for an Overweight Athlete who carries more than 20% body fat. He is trying to lose body fat as his primary goal, but also wants to maintain or increase his muscle mass. He weighs around 260 pounds and decides that he will shoot for around 2600 calories per day (260 x 10) as a starting point.

Baseline Meal Plan for a 260-pound male athlete trying to lose body fat AND maintain muscle.

Meal 1: 30 g complex carbohydrates/50 g protein/add 15 g healthy fats

½ cup oatmeal
Splenda for flavor
50 g whey protein
Handful almonds

Meal 2: 50 g protein/ add 15 g healthy fats/ vegetables
10 oz meat
Handful almonds
Veggies

Meal 3: 50 g protein/add 15 g healthy fats/ vegetables
10 oz meat
Handful almonds
Veggies

1 hr Pre-workout: 30 g complex carbohydrates/40 g protein
½ cup oatmeal
40 g whey protein

15 minutes pre-workout and throughout workout:
20 g BCAA
10 g glutamine
10g creatine

Meal 4: Post Workout: 30 g complex carbohydrates/50 g protein
½ cup oatmeal
Splenda
50 g whey

Meal 5: 50 g protein/ add 15 g healthy fats/green vegetables
10 oz meat
Salad with olive oil/vinegar as dressing

Meal 6: 50 g protein/ add 15 g healthy fats
1 scoop whey/ 1scoop casein or mixed protein blend with tbsp peanut butter

Totals:
2550 calories
300 g protein
100 carbohydrates
90 g fat
* Eat as many *green* veggies as you can and desire. Stay away from corn and carrots, unless you count them as your complex carbohydrate source. Vegetables in general will aid in stabilizing insulin levels, keep you full longer, and increase your overall health.

Macronutrient Manipulation to Reach Your Goals

So now we know where to start, and how many calories to begin our nutrition program with. We also better understand when to eat certain macronutrients to maximize our gains. But what if we want to get even bigger, leaner, or just tighten up? The answer lies in manipulating the amount of protein, carbohydrates, and fat we consume. As a general rule, never consume less than 1 gram of protein, per pound of body weight, per day. I actually prefer about 1.25-1.5 g/lbs/day but 1 g/lbs/day is a good rule. Likewise, healthy fats should never drop below 10% of your daily caloric intake. Carbohydrates are then the macronutrient we can manipulate to the greatest degree in pursuit of our goals.

So, whether we want to get bigger or leaner, greatly depends on our carbohydrate intake. We will realize greater gains in muscle mass and size if we increase complex carbohydrates. Likewise, if we want to lose body fat, reducing carbohydrates will significantly help in achieving our goal. A great place to start is with the 40/40/20 rule, then watch and see how your body reacts in relation to the goal you are after. If you want to get leaner or bigger, first start with a change in the amount of calories you consume. To start with, <u>**my caloric intake always changes by 160 calories, going up or down depending on my goal.**</u>

What If I Want To Get Leaner?

If I want to get leaner, I often decrease my carbohydrates by about 40 grams, which is around 160 calories (40 g x 4 calories/gram). If I do so though, I make sure my protein is at least 1g/lbs of bodyweight, and that fat is no less than 10% of my total calories. If this is not the case, then you must increase protein and fat accordingly.

As an example, if I am consuming 2600 calories of which 260 g is carbohydrates, I will drop that to 2440 calories and 220 g of carbohydrates. Then I'll monitor my progress. You may in fact find, as I have many times, that when you reduce carbohydrates you can increase protein by the same amount, and still lose body fat! This occurs in spite of the calorie totals being the same after the alteration. What!? If you decrease carbohydrates by 40 g, and increase protein by 40 g, how could you possibly lose body fat, don't both equal 4 calories per gram? Yes, but the answer lies in efficiency. Our bodies are able to use approximately 97% of the calories consumed when we eat carbohydrates. In contrast, when we eat protein, only 90% of the protein we consume is used! What happens to the rest? It is burned up as energy when we digest it. Remember, **protein actually burns more calories than the other macronutrients during digestion.**

Thus, in this case, if you find you feel weaker when you drop carbohydrates, or that you are losing muscle, just replace those calories with lean protein. Although your total calories will be the same, you still will lose body fat. This ensures that you are maintaining muscle, but storing less glycogen and fat with the reduced carbohydrate intake. With less glucose in the blood, and less glycogen stores in the muscle, fat is easier to tap into and burn. I believe losing more than 3 pounds per week signifies you are losing muscle. Two pounds is a great goal, and will ensure that you maintain the muscle you have worked so hard for. Skinny doesn't look good, its lean we are after, and the more muscle we carry, the more fat we'll burn!

What If I Want To Get Bigger?

Now, if I want to get bigger, I will increase my carbohydrates *and* protein in equal amounts. Once again I like to make a 160-calorie change, manipulating my carbohydrate and protein intake accordingly. In this case, it amounts to an addition of 20 g of protein and 20 g of carbohydrates, for a total of around 160 calories. I try this for two weeks and see how my body responds.

The following is a great example. Let's say I am consuming a total of about 260 g of carbohydrates on a 2600-calorie program. I also have set my goal to gain muscular weight. I realize after two weeks that I am losing weight. So, I make a change. No matter the goal, I always make a 160-calorie change in the amount of carbohydrates and protein I consume. This amount seems to make a difference, and will start you in the right direction. In this case, I want to get bigger, so unlike losing body fat, in which I would decrease *only* carbohydrates, I will do things a little different here. That is, still increase calories by around 160, but in the form of complex carbohydrates (20g) _and_ protein (20g). We can't just increase our lifting sessions, as over training can actually make us lose muscle. So when trying to gain mass, we must keep training hard, and increase our calories in the form of quality complex carbohydrates and protein.

So, I add 160 calories, which equals about 20 g of carbohydrates and 20 g of protein. I always add complex carbohydrates, rather than simple, to keep insulin stable and decrease fat accumulation. This bumps my total calories to 2750, with carbohydrates and protein at 280 g/day, and I see where I go from there. *This is by far the best way to gain quality muscle.* Once again, start with your baseline caloric intake, and increase accordingly with complex carbohydrates and protein.

As long as you are making progress towards the goals you set for yourself, you are accomplishing your task. It is very difficult to gain appreciable amounts of muscle without some fat gain. The body must be in a caloric surplus to gain a good deal of quality muscle. Remember, you must consume more than you burn to gain, and burn more than you consume to lose.

A Couple Commonly Asked Questions

Can you gain muscle while losing fat? Sure, although the process is slower. You also might notice that your weight stays very close to the same. It's the body composition that will change though, with fat being replaced by muscle. Watch the mirror!

Can you gain muscle on a low carbohydrate diet?
Sure, as long as protein and fats are increased enough to keep you in an anabolic, or growth phase. *Carbohydrates should never be completely excluded, and are vital around your workout period and breakfast.* Many make the mistake of eating whatever they want, gaining 20 pounds in one month, and thinking its all muscle. Wrong! Pay attention to how you look in the mirror as much as the scale. I believe photographs never lie, and believe them to be the best way to monitor progress. Skin calipers work, but in the wrong hands, can be more of a hindrance than help.

The Carbohydrate Cycle

The "Carbohydrate Cycle." Many bodybuilders and fitness professionals have used it throughout the years. I have used it to prepare for contests and many other times with great success. It can be a year round diet, or used to reach you goal of a lean, toned physique, no matter your sex.
The only thing I have found it not ideal for is gaining quality mass quickly. The reason is that you usually need a surplus of calories and carbohydrates to do this, and cannot worry about depleting glycogen by cutting carbohydrates. So, unless you are trying to gain 30 pounds of muscle this year, and just want to gain quality muscle while losing fat in the process, this program will work for you. I think most of us can handle that!

The Basics

The carbohydrate cycle is a combination of all we have discussed above. It is based on a system that allows you to vary your metabolism, taste buds, and glycogen levels. By doing these things, you will maximize fat loss while maintaining, and even adding muscle. Most of us would love to gain muscle at a slower but consistent rate while at the same time trimming body fat.

Nothing happens overnight, but in a matter of weeks, you will start to see major changes. Better than that, it is something you can follow year round and maintain without too much difficulty.

Now, we are not going to completely eliminate carbohydrates but rather cycle them. This will not only prevent all the negative qualities attributed to no carbohydrate diets, but it will also keep **leptin** levels from dropping too low. Again, leptin is a hormone that controls cravings and is greatly decreased when you drop carbohydrates or calories for too long. This will eventually cause us to go on binges and eat out of control, as the lower leptin levels drop, the greater hunger urges become. Not to mention depression, fatigue, and weakness that comes with not consuming enough carbohydrates. **The key then is to cycle between high and low carbohydrate consumption.** This not only fluctuates our metabolism, but allows leptin levels to slowly decrease for a few days while we burn fat, and then be replenished on our high carbohydrate days.

There are other benefits of cycling carbohydrates. After going on a low carbohydrate diet, many athletes feel as if they are losing muscle quickly. Most of the time though, it is an illusion. Water will follow carbohydrates into our muscles, thus causing them to appear full and pumped. When you go on a low carbohydrate program, the same water is pulled out of the muscle as the glycogen is spent, and you have the illusion of appearing smaller. The good news is that you body is more likely to rely on its fat stores when glycogen levels are low, and that is exactly what you want. Stay there too long though, and your fat burning will slow down considerably, not to mention psychologically feeling as if you are losing all your muscle.

Now, if you simply "carb" up every few days, the metabolism feels as if it has to pick up the pace to burn the extra calories you are consuming. By keeping your metabolism humming along, you will never plateau and continue to burn fat. Plus, when you "carb" up, you attain that "full" look again, and this can be great for the psyche. During a carbohydrate cycle, this can take place every few days.

I have found cycling carbohydrates to be very effective any time I am trying to lose body fat. In fact, I have often noticed that I have gained muscle while losing body fat on this program! It is not going to happen over night, but it can be done as long as you are consistent and work hard. Now, carbing up does not mean cheating, it simply means increasing your carbohydrates from complex, quality sources, once every few days. Once again, the basis of this diet is to vary your carbohydrate consumption to keep the gains coming without plateau.

Macronutrient Ratios

Protein intake should stay at least 1g/lbs/day, but will increase on low carbohydrate days. Healthy fat consumption should never drop below 10% and can go as high as 30%, once again on low carbohydrate days. The reasoning again is that both fats and carbohydrates are energy sources, and if one is reduced, we must combat that loss with another form of energy. I know it sounds counter intuitive, but the moderate consumption of healthy fats will not only aid in fat loss and muscle gains, but will provide energy lost from the carbohydrate reductions. High carbohydrate days should try to be scheduled on lifting days only. A great tip is **to never have two high carbohydrate days in a row.** Doing this may either add an excess amount of body fat or make you feel sluggish.

The advantages of carbohydrate cycles are:

1. Metabolic trickery-your body is continually changing its metabolism to counter the macronutrient and caloric fluctuations.

2. Tricking the body will allow it to "give up" extra fat for fuel when you take in less carbohydrates and calories.

3. You won't get bored with this program as you will be eating differently throughout the week.

4. It schedules the majority of your higher carbohydrate days for your toughest workouts.

5.   It restricts, or cuts out carbohydrates late at night to reduce fat accumulation. This is a great way to inhibit fat gains.

6. Cardio is still performed in the morning before your first meal. This ensures you get some carbohydrates after cardio, even on low days. It is always a good idea to take in BCAA and glutamine before cardio, no matter the day.

7. It provides faster and more consistent changes than any program I have tried. Better than that, the changes usually last, since this is not an "extreme diet" and can be maintained.

I will now outline two different carbohydrate cycles. Cycle one has more variability and seems to add a little more muscle to a physique, while cycle two favors those who want a more simplified approach. On cycle one, the week is divided into days of high, moderate, and low carbohydrate consumption. I usually go high on Tuesday and Sunday, medium on Monday, Thursday and Friday, and low on Wednesday and Saturday. I then repeat the cycle. Cycle two has 2-3 days of low carbohydrate consumption and then a high day. If I am on a deadline or getting very close, I usually have no cheat days, as I can't afford any setbacks at that time. But if I'm not, or feel I am far enough out, I feel cheat days are very important. It can keep you motivated, raise leptin levels, and gives you something to look forward to each week. It really all depends on the individual, current body fat, and goal in mind. That is why I usually schedule Sunday as a high day so if I decide to have a cheat day, I am not that far off what the day calls for.

Cycle 1

Cycle 1 is set up with three different splits. Your week is planned out having 2 high days, 2 low days and 3 medium days. NEVER have two high days back to back. Try to lift on high or medium days, and do cardio on low days. Following High days with Low or Low with High works the best!
High Carbohydrate Days: 2 days- <u>if you have a cheat day it counts as a high day</u>

Bodyweight (BW) x 1.5-1.75=carbohydrate in grams for the day
Bodyweight(BW) x 1= protein in grams for the day
Bodyweight (BW) x .25 = fat in grams for the day

- one piece of fruit allowed with each meal but NEVER after working out.
- Schedule at least one high day per week on leg day…you'll need it!
- Spread these out over 6-8 meals and try to get most of your carbohydrates before 7 PM

200 lbs individual would eat:

300-350 g carbohydrates
200 g protein
50 g fat

Approximately 2600 calories

Medium Carbohydrate Days: 3 days

Bodyweight (BW) x 1=carbohydrate in grams for the day
Bodyweight(BW) x 1.5= protein in grams fir the day
Bodyweight (BW) x .25 = fat in grams for the day

- One piece of fruit allowed at meal 1 and 2
- Spread these out over 6-8 meals and try to get most of your carbohydrates before 7 PM

200 lbs individual would eat:

200 g carbohydrates
300 g protein
50 g fat

Approximately 2450 calories

Low Carbohydrate Days: 2 days

Bodyweight (BW) x 0.5=carbohydrate in grams for the day
Bodyweight(BW) x 1.5= protein in grams for the day
Bodyweight (BW) x 0.35 = fat in grams for the day
•   No fruit allowed
•   Spread these out over 6-8 meals and try to get most of your carbohydrates before 3 PM

200 lbs individual would eat:

100 g carbohydrates
300 g protein
70 g fat
Approximately 2200 calories

Note:

1. ONE DAY PER WEEK- HAVE A CHEAT DAY OR MEAL…IF YOU DON'T HAVE A DEADLINE TO MEET!

2. Don't worry about calories, the correct amounts of grams taken in will equate to the right caloric intake.

Cycle 2

Cycle 2 is set up for those who like to follow the same protocol for a few days and then reward themselves. The low carbohydrate days are tough, but just remember a high carbohydrate day is right around the corner. Here is how Cycle 2 plays out:

- You will eat a low amount of carbohydrates on Monday and Tuesday with the only carbohydrates for breakfast, pre-, during, and post workout. Protein will be increased as will healthy fats.
- On Wednesday, your first priority with each meal is to get the amount of protein that you are scheduled to consume. Protein MUST be eaten first. Then you can have as many "quality" complex carbohydrates as you like with each meal.
- Thursday through Saturday you will repeat the same diet you followed on Monday and Tuesday. Sunday is a repeat of Wednesday and is ideal as you can get some cheat meals in there as it falls on Sunday...a great cheat day for football fans! I personally stay clean all week and if I want to, cheat on Sunday. You must be honest with yourself and remember what you are trying to accomplish.

On Low carbohydrate days (M, T, TR, F, S) consume...

- Protein- BW x 1.25-1.5
- Carbohydrates- BW x 0.5-0.6- No fruits allowed on low days
- Healthy Fats- BW x 0.25-0.37
- Eat as many green veggies as you want and don't count them in your totals.

- All these values are in grams and for a 200-pound athlete; this amounts to 250-300 g of protein, 100-120 grams of carbohydrates (ex. 30 for breakfast, 20 pre, 20 during the workout, 50 post workout), and 50-75g of healthy fats. That breaks down to about 30-40 g of protein per meal and 7-10 g of fat if you consume 8 meals. Don't worry about calories, the correct amounts of grams taken in will equate to the right caloric intake.

On High Carbohydrate days (Wednesday and Sunday) consume....

- Protein- BW x 1..Eat first!
- Carbohydrates- As many quality, complex sources as you wish and only eat until you are full. Don't stuff yourself until you feel like your going to pass out. Fruits are obviously allowed. Remember you have to eat your protein first!
- Fats- only that found in the food you eat.
- If you want to "cheat", only do so on a scheduled cheat day. This builds discipline and gives you something to look forward to. I prefer to schedule cheat meals on high days.
- Eat as many "green" veggies as you want and don't count them in your totals.
- All these values are in grams and for a 200 pound athlete, this amounts to 200 g of protein, unknown amount of carbohydrates and no extra healthy fats except that which is found in the food you are eating. That breaks down to about 25 g of protein per meal if you consume 8 meals. Make sure to get your protein down first. It will inhibit the insulin spike you will create when consuming all your carbohydrates as well as limit the amount of carbohydrates

you will eat. Remember, protein fills you up faster and prevents you from overeating. Once again, use common sense and I have found I rarely eat more than 300-350 g of carbohydrates on these high days.

- If you feel too weak or depleted on low days, then Cycle 1 or a baseline diet may be better for you. The low carbohydrate days are tough because you are forcing your body to burn fat and find other sources of energy. This is why the increased protein and healthy fat intake is a must to preserve muscle, keep you feeling full, and ensure adequate hormone production. Once again, you can gain muscle while inhibiting carbohydrates, as long as your healthy fat and protein amounts stay elevated. Don't worry about calories, the correct amounts of grams taken in will equate for the right caloric intake.

These two cycles are great examples of how to use carbohydrate manipulation to maximize your gains. There is no magic bullet or program here-it really is that simple. Don't worry about being 100% exact in regards to calories when you start these cycles. Just be consistent on your low and high days, and over time, your caloric intake will present itself. Write down your meal plans and try to get as close as you can. The key is to fluctuate your carbohydrates and calories-document all that you eat. This will allow you to make changes as needed, as well as document how you felt energy wise. Once again, notice protein and fat increased slightly on lower carbohydrate days. This is not a typo and is ideal. It will allow for a few more calories from protein and quality fats, which will keep you feeling full longer.

Try to refrain from lifting legs on lower carbohydrate days but rather focus on cardio. You will burn the most fat on these days as glycogen levels will be at their lowest. Schedule your toughest lifts for the higher carbohydrate days if you can. No matter the day, if you workout, take your BCAA, glutamine, and creatine as outlined earlier, along with your workout drinks comprised of fast digesting-high GI carbohydrates and whey protein. They are the most important meals of the day. This will ensure that your muscle is preserved and not lost. I suggest trying each of the three nutrition protocols outlined in this chapter, and find that which suits you best. Eventually you will be on your way to the physique you have always imagined.

Low Carbohydrate Mistakes

I put this section in to prevent many trainees from a mistake I have made many times. Cutting carbohydrates out completely. As you reduce carbohydrates on your off days, or during a carbohydrate cycle, you will notice the fat coming off quickly. This may lead to the thought, "Well, I will just stay away from carbohydrates all the time and eventually I will get the body I want." Wrong. Many trainers and individuals I know have tried prolonged low carbohydrate diets, as they seem to be the trend in today's market of quick fixes and 6-minute abs. While they may work in the beginning, they are by no means the right answer.

Why do they work? One of the reasons relates to hormones, as the insulin spike is far less pronounced when you reduce carbohydrate intake. This makes it less likely you will gain appreciable amounts of body fat. Glycogen levels are depleted, insulin levels remain low, and fat is used by the body to keep it running. Bodybuilders have been using low carbohydrate diets for many years, long before the recent trend. Also, nearly all of us have heard of the infamous Atkins diet. In fact, many of you reading this manual have probably found success on it. So, what's the problem and why am I so against it?

Well, to start with, while low carbohydrate programs work for a certain amount of time, they are by no means the long-term solution. Staying on such a diet to long is just not healthy. It can cause mood swings, depression and low energy levels. Glucose, or broken down carbohydrates, are after all the brains primary source of fuel. Another problem with cutting carbohydrates out completely is that you will probably put the weight back on one day. Why? It just isn't feasible to cut carbohydrates forever, and eventually you will snap, as leptin levels get too low and cravings become more insistent.

This is why carbohydrate cycles are such tremendous programs that can be used year round to reach your goals. They allow the benefits of reduced carbohydrates, but not for a prolonged period of time in which they can start to have negative effects. Who wants a great physique if we know eventually we will lose it again? The programs above will allow you to reap all the rewards of lower and higher carbohydrate days, as well maximize your muscle gains and fat loss.

In summary, first decide what you are trying to accomplish, and then chose a specific program to get you there. Some may chose to find their baseline caloric needs and make small fluctuations based on their goals. Others may decide to incorporate carbohydrate cycles to maximize their gains. In either case, I urge all of you to follow these tips in the pursuit of your transformation.

Water and Sleep

I won't ramble on and on about water and sleep. It is however an essential piece to the puzzle. If you are not adequately hydrated or rested, you will not be as successful in your transformation goals. Water and adequate rest not only aid in supporting our immunity and energy levels, but can affect the amount of fat we lose! If the body is in a state of dehydration or sleep deprivation, fat loss slows down as the body goes into more of a survival mode. Therefore, **try to drink at least a gallon of water per day and get 8 hours of sleep.** This means 128 ounces of fluid by the time you go to bed every night. Although you can drink diet soda, crystal light, ice tea, coffee, and any other calorie free beverages, I still prefer you drink 128 ounces of water per day. I love diet coke and drink my fair share, but also make sure to get a minimum of 128 ounces of water per day. Just drink 20 ounces with each meal, and you'll see it adds up fast. Get adequate amounts of sleep, drink your water, and you'll continue to make positive changes. These simple things can make all the difference in the world.

Important Note:

Please **DO NOT** drink a gallon of water at one sitting!!! Drinking an excessive amount of water all at once, or even over the course of the day can cause serious health issues and even death. Spread your water intake evenly throughout the day and if you're thirsty, by all means drink! Just don't try to make up for a "busy" day by drinking all 128 ounces at once. You are only asking for trouble.

Cheat Days

I often refer to taking a cheat meal or day throughout this chapter. I really think it is vital to keep you sane, make sure you don't get burned out, and satisfy your cravings. If you don't want too, or have a strict deadline to meet, by all means, stay the course. I just don't want you to think that by taking one cheat day a week that all your success will be lost. Many times it can be a good thing as you satisfy what you have been holding out on all week, as well as mixing up your metabolism. Some have even told me that cheating one day a week helps them remember what it felt like to eat lousy. After that, it's easy to get back on course. Believe me, it takes more than one day to completely derail all your hard work, although it may feel like you gained 20 pounds in one day! Often it is just glycogen stores filling back up along with water retention. Remember, water follows glycogen. Cheating usually isn't a good thing in life, but in this case, it can keep you on the road to your goals. Be smart, but don't fear cheat days-you earned it!

Nutrition Summary

Rule 1: Be consistent in your nutrition-cheating 4 days per week will never get you where you want to be.

Rule 2: Know that nutrition is responsible for 75% of what you look like.

Rule 3: Never consume less than 1 g of protein/lbs/day and less than 10% of your caloric intake from healthy fats-no matter what program you follow. Carbohydrates are the most adjustable macronutrient.

Rule 4: Time your nutrients to maximize muscle gains.

- Consume Complex carbohydrates and lean protein at most meals.
- Consume the majority of your carbohydrates at breakfast and surrounding your workout.
- Consume BCAA, glutamine, and creatine before and after workouts-this includes cardio!
- Consume a drink mix during your lifting sessions made of simple carbohydrates, glutamine, creatine and BCAA.
- Consume Whey Protein and fast digesting carbohydrates post workout.
- Reduce carbohydrates at night unless post workout (vegetables are the exception)
- Have a casein protein source with healthy fats as your last meal before bed.

Rule 5: Consume your daily caloric intake over 6-8 meals, and try to drink 20 ounces of water with each meal. This will allow you to drink a gallon of water per day, which greatly increases fat loss, immunity and overall health. Also, don't forget to get adequate rest.

Rule 6: As a general rule-take bodyweight x 12-15 to get starting caloric intake. Lower or raise that value depending on your goals, activity level, and how you are progressing.

Rule 7: On a baseline program-start with approximately 40% carbohydrates, 40% protein, and 20 % healthy fats to make up your baseline caloric intake.

Rule 8: When trying to get leaner or bigger, make 160-calorie adjustments in your caloric intake. Reduce complex carbohydrates when trying to lean out, and increase complex carbs and protein when trying to gain mass. Do this until you start moving in the right direction, and give each change two weeks to see if it's working.

Rule 9: One of the best nutrition protocols for natural bodybuilders and athletes is to use carbohydrate cycles. It is the ideal way in my opinion to make the most significant changes in your physique.

Rule 10: Unless you are on a deadline-take one cheat day a week. It will motivate you to work hard the entire week and keep you focused. **Rarely is one day responsible for a poor physique.**

Don't Forget....:

To get Lean: Expend more than you Consume

To gain Mass: Consume more than you Expend

Good Luck!

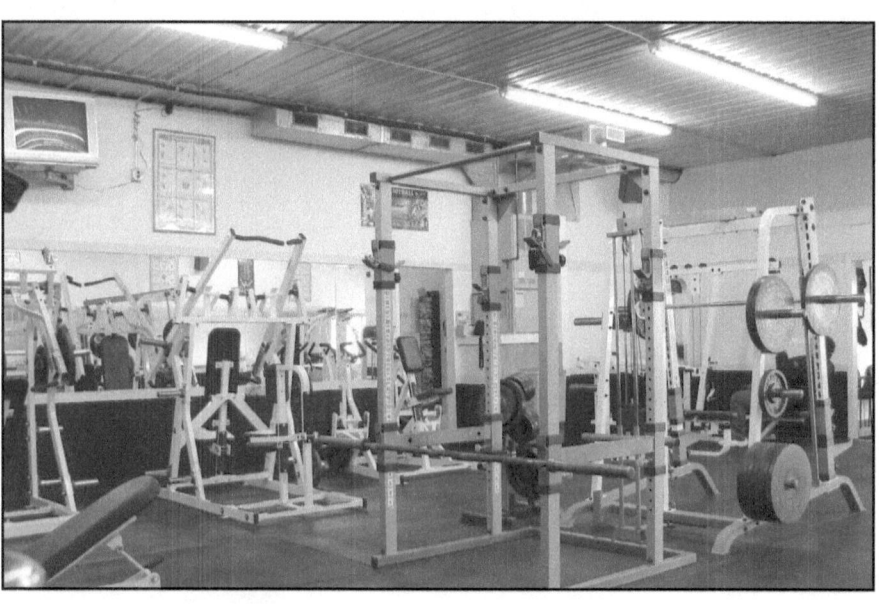

Chapter 6

TRAINING: THE EIGHT PRINCIPLES

Here we go, the chapters that finally puts it all together, with the topic many probably wished I had started with-training. We have covered hormones, nutrition, nutrient timing, diets, and supplementation. In these final pages, I will discuss training protocols and how to maximize any training program you follow. The final chapters also include some of my favorite programs on nutrition, cardio, and weight training. Although these workouts have worked well for me, you may have to make small adjustments suited towards your specific needs. I find it very frustrating to read workout after workout, each claiming to be the magic bullet. The truth is, no such workout or program exists, only time tested principles and techniques tailored to each individual.

The principles that we are about to discuss should always be present in your workout programs. If you practice these principles and consistently re-evaluate your goals, you will be successful. Although I change my workouts constantly, *I always practice the principles you are about to learn.* Along with solid nutrition and supplement protocols, you will see more gains and positive changes in your physique than you ever imagined. Should the programs I use not suit your goals or comfort level, I promise, the ideal program for you exists! In fact, with the principles and information presented in this chapter, *you* will be able to create the ideal program suited to your individual needs. That, after all, is true mastery. Now, before we can discuss training though, we must fully understand what we are trying to change in the first place, the muscles themselves.

Fast and Slow

Generally speaking, the muscles have two main fibers, type I (slow twitch) and type II (fast twitch). Slow twitch are generally considered **endurance or aerobic (with oxygen) fibers**, while fast twitch are generally considered **strength or anaerobic (without oxygen) fibers**. As an example, sprinters rely more on fast twitch fibers while marathon runners rely more on slow twitch. Fast twitch fibers have various subtypes (IIa, IIb, IIc)-some having higher endurance (IIa), and others having lower endurance but better strength potential (IIb/IIc). Slow twitch fibers have subtypes as well, all having high endurance and low strength capabilities. In any case *type II fibers are most responsible for muscular growth and are what we should primarily focus on* (Fig 11).

Fig. 11

Type I (mostly aerobic): Slow Twitch-High Endurance-Poor Size Potential

Type II (mostly anaerobic): Fast Twitch-Low/Moderate Endurance-Excellent Size Potential

- Type **IIa-highest endurance/lowest strength potential of type II**

- Type **IIb-moderate endurance/moderate strength potential**

- Type **IIc-lowest endurance/greatest strength potential of type II**

Note: very small percentage of our muscle fibers are made up of IIc

Muscle, when stimulated by a weight, generally calls upon these fibers in a specific order. The slow twitch-type 1 fibers are first to fire with their higher aerobic capacity and low strength potential. This makes sense as at the beginning of most sets we are fresh and the weights seem easy. As the set continues the muscles then engage the type IIa fibers, the more aerobic of the fast twitch subtypes. Still, these fibers carry much more strength potential than type I. Finally as the weights get very heavy, oxygen decreases, lactic acid builds up, and we can barely get another rep, the muscles fire their highest threshold anaerobic fast twitch fibers, generally IIb, IIc and the remainder of IIa. *It is the stimulation of these high threshold fibers than can make or break our muscle gains.*

To trigger stimulation of these higher threshold fibers, we must challenge our muscles and push them to the point of failure. The weights must be challenging, but must *also stimulate as many fibers as possible to maximize our gains.* Should you lift an extremely heavy weight for low reps, the type IIc and IIb fibers will be called upon quickly and most often, but the CNS will shut down long before the muscle is fully taxed. We will explain that soon, but in the case of low reps and quick sets, strength is often the goal, as the muscles aren't stimulated long enough to maximize their growth potential. Should you do very high rep sets, say 30 _easy_ reps with a very light weight, type I and IIa will get the majority of the stimulation, with type IIb and IIc fibers not being stimulated much at all (Fig. 12). Once again, we didn't stimulate all fibers properly as the high threshold fibers will get little stimulation.

Fig. 12 Muscle fibers are called upon to perform specific tasks.

Lift Heavy Weight/Low Reps/Low Endurance→Favor Type IIb and IIc

Lift Light Weight/High Reps/High Endurance→ Favor Type I and some IIa

The longer the set and lighter the resistance, the more the endurance fibers will be stimulated, such as type IIa and I. The heavier the weight, the more stimulation type IIb and IIc will get. Again, to gain the most muscle and maximize our physique, *we must stimulate all fibers with an emphasis on the highest threshold type II fibers.* How do we accomplish this-aren't some more endurance oriented and others more strength oriented? How could we possibly do both? There are a few tricks to make sure we hit all these fiber types and the first is increased **time under tension.**

This refers to how long there is continuous tension on the muscle during a set. While increasing time under tension works extremely well, we can also accomplish the same thing by incorporating extended set techniques such as drop sets, x-reps, super sets and multi-rep rest-pause training (we will discuss these soon!). Even though there is a brief pause between some of these techniques it is minimal at best. In any case, if the set lasts long enough, and the resistance is adequate, the muscles will be called upon in a domino-like fashion *until those most responsible for growth are stimulated*. They will have no choice!

The longer you can sustain your set *__past the initial stimulation of these high threshold fibers,__* the more gains you will see. Studies have shown that sustaining your set for at least 30seconds can greatly enhance stimulation of *all muscle fibers*, specifically the high threshold growth fibers. If your set is only 15 seconds long, then time under tension will not be sufficient for maximum growth and our muscular gains will fall short. What will happen in this case is a termination of your set **before** the high threshold fibers are adequately stimulated.

Many resistance programs call for reps in the 8-12 range and for good reason. In this case, the slow twitch fibers will be stimulated first, followed by the low threshold- fast twitch fibers, and finally the high threshold growth fibers. Things are easy to start with, which is why the aerobic-slow twitch fibers are activated first. As the set progresses and oxygen supply to the muscle decreases, the more anaerobic fast twitch fibers are called into play. **It isn't until the last few reps that the highest threshold type II's are activated**. That is why the last few reps are so crucial, as they will tap into the high threshold fibers most responsible for growth. The problem with many is that they only complete 1-2 reps once these high threshold fibers are activated and thus fail to grow much.

Again, this is why increased TUT is so important, as many individuals don't get enough stimulation of the high threshold fibers to initiate growth. Their sets end before these fibers are **forced** to wake up, and it is these high threshold fibers that are most responsible for growth. The longer you can stimulate them, the more successful you will be. Sure, if you lift with an extremely heavy weight, you'll quickly tap into the high threshold fibers, but the time you sustain this set usually only lasts 10-15 seconds and the nervous system is taxed more than the muscle. In fact the most recent research is showing that even longer tension times, in excessive of 50 seconds, can dramatically increase muscle growth!

Are you starting to see why so many people year in and year out never acquire more muscle? They do 3 sets of 8 reps, with the same weight, but complete each set in 15 seconds or less. This once again isn't long enough to trigger the maximum growth response, at least not in the majority of the population. Sure, some individuals can tap very quickly into all their fibers, and therefore find success with typical 6-10 rep sets lasting 15-20 seconds. They go through the continuum very quickly and stimulate the high threshold fibers with ease. Most of us aren't that lucky though, and have to push a little harder at the end of most sets to tap into these growth fibers. So how do we do this, how do we lift for a longer period of time, *with* challenging weights, to get at these high threshold growth fibers? The weight can't be too light or the high thresholds won't be activated. It can't be too heavy or the set will terminate very quickly. **The answer lies in extended set techniques or high volume protocols.** We will start with the latter.

High Volume vs Extended Set Techniques

High volume entails performing a high number of sets (>15), which eventually exhausts all fibers types. While tension is released from the muscle between sets, the high number of sets eventually taps into all the fibers. *This in my opinion is not ideal though*, as it can lead to over-training and injury. I prefer to use a lower number of sets with **extended set techniques** such as drop sets, x-reps, multi-rep rest pause training and super sets to get to these high threshold fibers. _These techniques allow you to extend your sets and maximize growth with a much lower volume_.

If I Want to....Does High Volume Work?

Let's look at high volume a little closer. What if you did high volume workouts, such as 20 sets of 10 reps, would it work? Well, you would definitely hit all the fiber types, work the endurance and strength components, and initiate growth, but also spend many hours in the gym, inhibit recovery time, and increase joint pain. There is much debate out there as to which is better: high volume vs. low volume. Again, high volume refers to a large number of sets, usually 15 or more, while low volume is usually performed with sets in the 6-12 range.

I will be honest and say that 75% of the time, I shy away from high volume and prefer low volume with extended set techniques. We will discuss these techniques later but I will say that both high and low volume have their merits. Some individuals feel they must do 15 sets of barbell curls to make gains. Others feel they can do 3 very intense sets and make the same progress. Both protocols will eventually hit the fast twitch fibers and induce growth. You must however whey your ability to recover with the number of set you perform, body type, risk of injury, and confidence in your program. I will discuss more on why I feel low volume/high intensity work is best, but if you love high volume workouts, don't worry, they do have their place and can be used.

Increase the Resistance

The next technique we'll touch on is called **progressive overload**, which is also critical to making gains. This technique focuses on the principle; *that we must continually increase the workload on the muscle to force growth and strength increases*. If you lift with the same weight over the course of weeks and months, why would the muscle keep growing stronger? It won't, it will only adapt to the given stimulus and then stabilize. Power lifter's use progressive overload quite often, and is one of the reasons they get stronger, as well as more muscular over time. They focus on progressively increasing the workload with each set, and while they often hit failure very quickly, the high volume of sets they perform can often stimulate a great deal of fibers. These athletes are geared more towards training their nervous systems to adapt to heavier weights, and could care less about fiber stimulation as long as they keep getting stronger. For most of us, muscular gains follow strength increases in a stair step pattern. Essentially, strength goes up linearly while size follows behind and occurs in spurts. So in the case of power lifters, muscular gains are often a side effect of they're progressive, high volume training protocols that increase strength.

Lesson Learned?

The lesson we can take from power lifters then is if one wishes to gain muscle, we must first get stronger. While power lifters are amazing athletes and do get stronger and more muscular, they don't often attain the "balanced" physique of those who use a mixture of increased TUT *and* progressive overload. While I believe progressive overload is vital if you want to get more muscular, we need to also incorporate increased TUT to maximize other avenues of muscle growth. Not only does increasing TUT stimulate the high threshold fibers, but also increases blood flow and capillary expansion in the muscle. So the point is, *we shouldn't sacrifice other techniques that can lead to muscle growth and better aesthetics.* Rather, we should use *all* techniques to maximize every route we can towards making gains.

So we now know that when trying to build muscle, we need to hit the fast twitch fibers more frequently and for a longer period of time. We also know we must progressively increase the resistance. What about rep ranges, should we focus on reps in the low range, 1-5, or high range, 8-15? Let's find out.

Low Reps or High Reps?

Numerous studies have shown the greatest strength gains occur in the 1-5 rep range, and the most muscular gains occur in the 8-12 rep range. Lifting for strength will eventually lead to muscular growth, but again, it will come in spurts. Why not have your cake and eat it too? By working both the strength and tension/endurance components, you can stimulate all fibers and maximize your growth potential. We will discuss how to incorporate both into your training as this chapter unfolds, but for now, realize you can stimulate and build the most muscle by:

1. Progressively increasing your weights

2. Extending tension times

3. Varying your rep ranges

Don't Do High Volume with High Intensity!

Again, I think doing the same amount of work in less time is the way to go, but I do occasionally mix in high volume workouts to add variability to my training. A great example is the legendary German Volume Training (GVT). GVT has been around for ages and refers to taking 60% of your one-rep-max on one specific lift, performing 10 sets of 10 reps, with minimal rest periods, *all with the same weight!* **This is the only exercise you do for that body part.** Even though you're not increasing the weight, in some ways you are, as you must attempt to get 10 reps each time! It is brutal but highly effective, and by the end, 60% feels like 200%! In this case, you are increasing the resistance by forcing yourself to get 10 reps each set, and the high threshold fibers will be adequately stimulated secondary to the high volume.

The one thing an individual should be cautious about is high volume with extended set techniques. *In this case, drop sets, x-reps, and other advance techniques are absolutely contraindicated.* What I mean is, if you prefer multiple sets with multiple reps, you shouldn't use techniques such as drop sets and supersets. This leads to nothing but over-training and injury, and can keep you out of the gym for a long time. That is exactly why I prefer shorter, more intense workouts.

Is It That Simple?

Now, if all we have to do is increase the time under tension, lift progressively heavier weights, and vary our rep ranges, then why read on? Well, it is because the body has a set of rules it lives by and could care less if you want to build the body you want. The body's simple purpose in life is to make sure we don't hurt ourselves and survive. So, when a lifter fails at the end of a set with a heavy weight, it often isn't because he doesn't "want" to lift it, but rather because the "mind-muscle" connection fails long before the muscle is ready to quit. This is to "protect" the muscle, as the brain realizes the severe stressor and will just not allow the muscle to go on. Think of it as the brain being the parents that just won't let their kids go out on a rainy day to play. It is for their own good, and the brain is doing the same, or so it thinks, by inhibiting the contraction of a muscle past a certain number of reps or weight limit. The downside is that when this "shut down" occurs, the muscle usually hasn't been under a state of continuous tension, at least not long enough, to initiate the maximum growth response. Once again, it is the body's way of protecting itself. The brain realizes the stressor and just stops sending signals to the muscle long before it is ready to quit.

Neuromuscular Efficiency

This process of "self-protection" we just discussed is related to **neuromuscular efficiency.** Neuromuscular efficiency simply refers to how efficiently our brain can stimulate our muscles to act. The central nervous system (CNS=brain and spinal cord) controls everything that we do. So, when our muscles are stimulated to lift a weight, our brain has to send a signal **strong enough** to move that weight. Remember though that our brain and body are essentially made to protect us. So, when a weight we start to lift stimulates our muscles, the brain has to decide whether it should push forward, or inhibit any more nerve impulses to the muscle.

This easily explains why an individual progresses so quickly when they first started lifting. The communication between the muscle and CNS became more efficient as more fibers were stimulated with each increase in weight and training session. Initially, since few were stimulated in the absence of training, it was easy to wake up a few muscle fibers and initiate growth and strength increases. *Then, as the weights got heavier, we started to fail.* This simply happened because there weren't enough nerve-muscle communications stimulated to complete the contraction and keep us progressing. Soon we became frustrated and either stopped working out, or did the same weights repeatedly. Hence, the body ceased to change anymore.

Now, with prolonged and progressive training, using various techniques such as increased TUT and progressive overload, the "mind-muscle" connection learns to become more in sync, and more weight can be lifted. There are those of course who we have deemed "naturally strong and muscular," and these individuals simply have tremendous "mind-muscle" connections to start with. You know, the guy who weighs 200 pounds, can bench press 400 pounds, and only does 6-10 reps once per week! The point is they can summon a tremendous amount of nerve-muscle connections very easily, get to the "growth" fibers quickly, and thus stimulate their muscles to grow with minimum sets and reps.

Most of us are not that lucky. For most, including myself, the brain will deem a weight to large for the amount of muscle we have, and it forces us to stop by not allowing us to complete any more repetitions. So, it inhibits the response sent to the muscle, and we therefore can't lift a given weight load. This is called **CNS shut down**. It is a process in which the CNS will "shut down" muscle contraction long before the muscle is fully stimulated. It is once again done to protect our muscles from stress and damage, but is **one of the main reasons so many of us fail to gain muscle, as the high threshold fibers are not adequately stimulated.**

You must understand this, so you can recognize when this occurs, and change your training accordingly. It is important to realize that the muscle and CNS are different. Our muscles need that progressive overload and extended tension time to initiate the growth response. The muscle has its own "needs" and if the CNS shuts down before the muscle meets the stimulus it needs to grow, it just simply won't! So, what techniques are we going to use to increase the TUT and get past CNS shutdown? How can we continue to make strength and muscle gains if our CNS shuts down long before we want it to? That is exactly what the next section is all about!

Understanding the Mind-Muscle Connection

To review, when it comes to contraction of a muscle, the signal begins in the brain and then travels to the spinal cord. From there it travels to the peripheral nerves and then terminates at the muscle. Now, to take it step further, when a nerve approaches a muscle it actually splits into many tiny branches with each one supplying a number of muscle fibers. We call this interaction a **motor unit.** *A motor unit is essentially the combination of the nerve branch and the muscle fibers it supplies* (Fig 13). The body does not activate all its available motor units when we lift a weight. In fact, it tries to protect us by firing as few motor units as possible to get the job done. The lighter the weight, the lower the threshold, and the less motor units stimulated. As an example, there are less motor units fired when we pick up a glass of water versus when we lift a 40-pound dumbbell. The trick then is _forcing_ the body to activate more motor units, which will then lead to increased strength and muscular gains. Exactly what we are trying to accomplish.

Fig 13.

When a weight is lifted, the stimulus is sent to the brain, and from there, it must decide how many motor units it will "call" upon to act. To get stronger and more muscular, we must awaken more motor units as the weights increase.

	Resistance Lifted	Motor Units (nerves + muscle)
	Light weight	Some motor units activated (low threshold)
CNS----→ (brain + spinal cord)	Moderate weight	More motor units activated (med. threshold)
	Heavy Weight	Large number of motor units activated
		(HIGH THRESHOLD)

Adaptations

Since the brain controls how many motor units fire, it doesn't matter how many muscle fibers you have if the signal doesn't activate enough of them. The muscle is useless without its nerve branch, and vice versa, as together they make up the motor unit. So, with intense training and various techniques, we **teach** our brain to activate more motor units, thus stimulating more muscle and lifting more weight.

Now, as stated before, there are specific adaptations that occur that prohibit us from lifting more. If we understand them, we can overcome them, and continue to make gains. The first thing the body does when a stimulus (lifting a weight) is induced is to make sure it doesn't sustain an injury. So if you are trying to curl a barbell, the body will actually use the tricep to oppose the lift. It is called an agonist/antagonist relationship. As you lift more and more frequently, the antagonist or opposing muscle begins to relinquish, and you aren't as inhibited in your lift. The take home point here is that the *more you train, the less opposition your target muscle will sustain from its antagonist, and the more motor units you can fire.* **This is the first adaptation.** The **second adaptation** is *how quickly the motor units will fire once stimulated.* The more you train, the quicker they'll fire and the stronger you'll be. The **third and final adaptation** is *increasing the amount of time these motor units can sustain their increased firing rate.* Obviously, it is one thing to fire additional motor units more quickly, but it is even more beneficial to fire them for a longer period of time. These three adaptations, brought about with proper training, will vastly improve the "mind-muscle connection."

Now that we have talked about how the muscles and nervous system interact, we can manipulate the system to our benefit. What we must understand, again, is that the nervous system is one of our greatest inhibitors of growth. It just doesn't want us to get hurt or build more metabolically expensive muscle. *The only way we will grow then is to inhibit the CNS from stopping our muscle gains and force the body to change.* Even by increasing the activation of more motor units, as well as the rate and duration of firing, the CNS will still die out before the muscle is ready to quit. So we need to find a way to keep the muscle stimulated long after the CNS fatigues. This will ensure that the high threshold motor units, those most responsible for growth, are fully stimulated by weight and tension times.

Satellite Cells

I am not going to bore you much longer but an important point I want to touch on are **satellite cells.** These are the actual cells responsible for building more muscle. We aren't necessarily trying to create these cells, as they are always present along most muscle fibers. What we are trying to do though is "convince" them into differentiating and fusing with existing muscle fibers. **That's when the muscle building process occurs.** Once we initiate a stimulus great enough, such as lifting weights, GH and IGF-1 are produced, and these satellite cells "wake up" and fuse with existing, traumatized muscle fibers. Thus, initiating the muscle building process.

This is physiologically one of the ways in which we build and repair our muscle tissue, along with all the nutritional and supplement protocols we have touched on. As I am sure you know by now, "conventional" tactics won't trigger the greatest hormone or satellite cell response. The stimulus must be great enough, and long enough, for the body to summon these cells and initiate the rebuilding process. If it isn't, they will lie dormant, and building muscle will be more difficult.

How Do We Actually Do All This?

So how do we get past CNS failure, lift progressively heavier weights, increase time under tension, and initiate the greatest satellite cell and hormone response? Well, for starters, we have to be honest with ourselves. Many of us stop when we can't lift another rep, and if we do this, it is usually at the point in which only some of our muscle fibers are fatigued. By extending the set and using advanced techniques, we can stimulate the last few fibers most responsible for increased muscular gains. This will produce more hormones, activate more satellite cells and motor units, as well as get past CNS limitations.

Building an Effective Program

"If you want what you've never had, you must do what you've never done."

-Anomymous

So, where do we start? What training methods do we use? If you think about it, the countless magazines and books out there provide enough different workout schemes to last a lifetime. If you look close though, the ones that work all have a few things in common. I call them the **Eight Principles Of Resistance Training.**

1. High Intensity

2. Increased Time Under Tension

3. Progressive Overload

4. Blood Flow and Occlusion

5. The Negative

6. Stretch

7. Variability

8. Time Off

High Intensity:

You must train with intensity.

To start with, we first and foremost have to train with intensity. If you don't, you are only cheating yourself. There are 168 hours in a week and you definitely can give up a few hours for lifting and cardiovascular training. By training hard and really pushing ourselves to the max, we *will* make gains. Gains lead to confidence and confidence keep us going. We must treat each workout, each rep, and each week as a chance to get better. Intensity is needed to push past previous plateaus and keep our body from stabilizing. Push hard and challenge yourself.

If you want to succeed and see major changes, you will have to suffer. Taking yourself to a place you rarely go, physically and mentally, is often needed to cause a growth response or a loss of body fat. It isn't fun at the time but once your done you will truly feel you have accomplished something. Remember, the body loves stability and the stimulus must be great enough to initiate change. Go in there and tell yourself that you will do better than the last time, no matter what. We only have so many workouts left in our life and each one lost is one we will never get back.

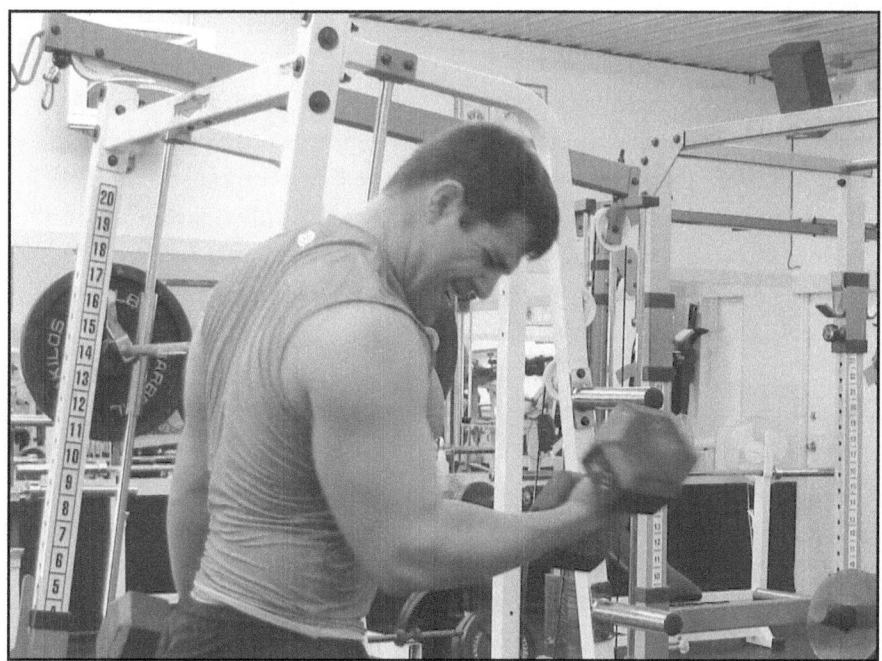

Intensity- With intense workouts and persistence you can achieve your goals.

No matter the program you decide to follow, it is key to maintain your focus and intensity. You can ease up during the time off phase and actually need to. At all other times though you should workout intensely and with a purpose.

Increased Time Under Tension (TUT):

You must extend your set to the point in which the high threshold fibers are stimulated.

We touched quite a bit on this earlier, but increased TUT is one of the most overlooked aspects in resistance training. Studies have shown numerous times that to maximize stimulation of the high threshold growth fibers you must extend your set *past positive muscle failure*. This can be accomplished through continuous tension on the muscle for 30-50 seconds, or with the use of super sets, x-reps, drop sets, or other techniques. From what I have observed in the gyms I have trained in, the average set lasts 15-20 seconds, half of what is most conducive to growth. It is a vital component, and you'll see why soon.

Many individuals do 3 sets of 8 reps and if you time them, you may get a time under tension of 12-15 seconds, not even half of what you need! Now, there may be times when strength gains are your goal and muscle growth is not. While this will have a time and a place in our training protocol, it won't be ideal all the time. In building strength we are more focused on neuromuscular efficiency. Activating more motor units with each training session. In this case, time under tension is low, which means you may get stronger but not bigger, as the CNS adapts to the stimulus. The muscle however is not stimulated to grow nearly as efficiently as with increased tension times.

Sure, as we touched on before, in time you will get bigger as strength has been said to increase linearly and size in a stair step pattern. I have noticed such changes personally with my strength continuing to increase while my muscle size did not. Then over the course of two weeks, I seemed to see major changes. This is called the principle of progressive overload and we will discuss that soon. For now, realize that to maximally stimulate muscle growth, we must ensure that time under tension is sufficient, and that we fully stimulate the high threshold growth fibers.

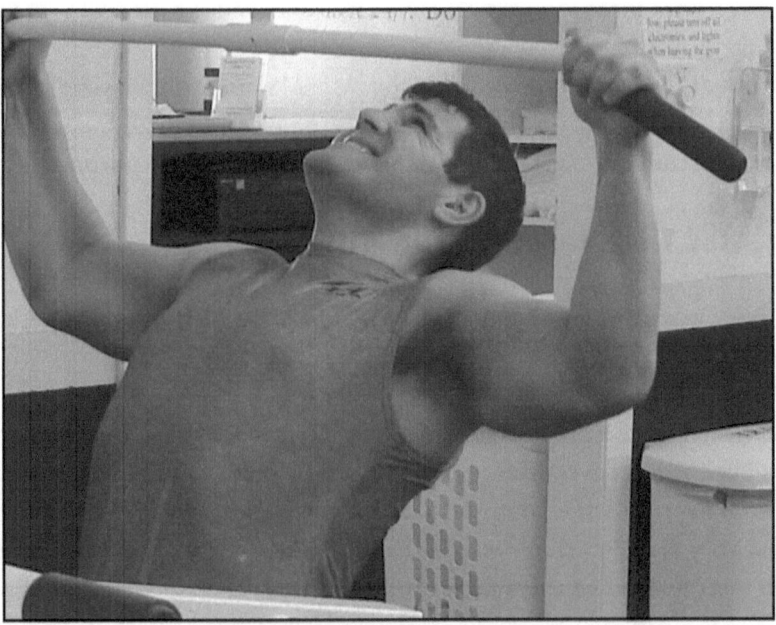

Extending your set to the point in which the high threshold motor units are stimulated is essential to maximize your gains.

Jonathan Lawson and Steven Holman from Iron Man magazine invented the technique called **X Reps** and it has changed the way I, and many others are lifting. In the past, many bodybuilders have used the term partials to describe this technique. What this entails is to complete a set of a given exercise, as specified by your program, and then when you reach neuromuscular failure (can't do another rep), you continue with 8-10 inch pulses in the semi-stretched position. This basically is the location in the lifts range of motion in which the muscle is under maximum tension and has its greatest power potential. You can do them at any range during the lift but the most effective is the semi-stretched position.

Lets take cables curls. When you can't do another full range rep, you lift the weight to the spot where you can't get it any higher, lower 8 inches under constant tension, back up to the stop point, back down, etc. until you can't move the weight at all. This will give you another 15 seconds of stimulation and keep the muscle firing to illicit a greater growth response _past_ CNS shutdown. This removes, or reduces the effect of CNS failure that is preventing you from getting another full rep, and it all occurs after you reach positive failure. You know, the point where you usually stopped before! It is an intense technique and is very difficult, physically and mentally. The effects are mind blowing though and for more information on this amazing technique go to www.x-rep.com and purchase some of their e-books. They are some of the best I have ever read.

There are other ways to increase the time under tension and maximize fiber recruitment. A few of my favorites are drop sets, super sets and multi-rep rest pause techniques. **Drop sets** are essentially two sets of the same exercise repeated back to back without rest. On the second set, the weight is usually dropped 20-30% and the set is continued. For instance, if you were doing bench presses with 225 pounds for 8 reps and then hit failure, you would quickly reduce the weight to perhaps 185 pounds and continue immediately to failure. **Super sets are** usually two different exercises, completed back to back without rest. **Multi-rep rest-pause training** is described as taking a given weight that would produce maximum failure at 8-10 reps. At the eighth to tenth rep, when you hit 100% failure, you put the weight down, rest 15-20 seconds and resume with the same weight. This time you more than likely will only get 4-6 reps. After you fail on this rep range, you rest another 15-20 seconds. Finally, you end by completing one final set with the same weight, usually getting 1-2 reps. This technique is brutal and will tax all your fast twitch fibers. I often use this technique and add X-reps to the end of it. The combinations are endless!

The key here is that there is very little if any rest between sets on all the protocols we just described. That allows all muscle fibers (slow to fast) to be fully stimulated. Believe me, this is not something to be taken lightly as these techniques with tax you mentally and physically.

Summary of Advanced Techniques:

X-Reps or partials: It is essentially a continuation of any set, on any exercise, after positive failure is reached. After you can no longer complete a full rep, focus on the 8-10" range of motion where tension is maximal, usually the mid point of any lift. Continue performing as many reps as possible in 8-10" pulses until you can't even do that anymore! Go to www.x-rep.com to learn more about this revolutionary technique. Some have referred to these as partials in the past.

Drop Sets: two sets of the <u>**same exercise**</u> repeated back to back without rest. There is a 20-30% reduction of weight for the second set.

Super Sets: two <u>**different exercises**</u>, completed back to back without rest.

Multi-Rep Rest Pause: Take a given weight that you can get 8-10 reps to failure, rest 15-20 seconds, then repeat with the same weight until failure (usually 4-6 reps), again rest 15-20 seconds and finish with one last set to failure (1-2 reps). This amounts to a total of 14-20 reps with the same weight.

Now, drop sets, supersets, and partials are not the only way to hit all fiber types. Although I believe they are the most efficient, you can set up a program to focus on high volume (many sets) if you wish. I firmly believe that you don't ever need more than 12 sets per body part, but confidence in your program is key. Therefore, if you feel you need more sets, then by all means perform them. Many athletes, such as the great Bill Pearl and

Arnold, felt that they needed a high volume workout to initiate gains. These would often include 20-25 sets per body part. I would rather have an athlete train on a program they believe in than train with one they don't. If you need 15-20 sets to make gains that's fine, just limit the use of drop sets, x reps and super sets. I promise this will lead to over training and injury if combined with excessively high volume.

What Set-Up Do I Use?

Personally, I change workouts frequently but usually focus on 6-12 sets per body part and incorporate extended set techniques often. There are times when I train with volume, but these are few and far between, and only to shock my system into growing again. Variability is key and sometimes a shock to the system is all it takes to restart the growth process. The programs I use most frequently are set up with a variety of rest periods, reps, weights, and exercises, but we'll review that later. For now, understand that it takes various techniques to get past CNS failure, hit all fiber types, and initiate the growth process. Remember, muscle is a privilege and we have to work hard for it.

Progressive Overload:

You must strive to get stronger with each workout.
This is one of the most important aspects of strength training and body transformation. We briefly touched on it earlier when discussing power lifters and it is one of the major reasons they have large amounts of dense musculature, even when their time under tension is reduced. This principle simply states; you must make progress each week, on the first set, of each exercise you perform. In most cases, it is with a compound lift and the goal is to generate maximum force with each rep. If you lifted 225 for 8 reps the week before, you must do 225 x 9 reps this week. You must challenge the muscles and force them to change. If the stimulus remains the same, so will the body. Why wouldn't it? Remember, the body will have to work extra hard to support all that new muscle and unless it is forced to produce it, it won't. I know because I made that mistake for years. I would train with intensity, but with the same weights and the same workouts. Guess what, I hardly changed at all.

We must initiate a stimulus, progressively more difficult, with each workout. This is where many athletes screw up. They do the same workout, with the same weights, each week. The body may change initially but it will eventually cease to progress. By providing a more difficult stimulus each workout, we will force the body and muscles to change. The body must think, "Hey, this guy means business, if we don't make some changes we are in trouble!" Thus, the muscle begins to change in response to the stimulus by growing bigger and stronger.

Simply stated, **you will not increase muscle mass or get leaner if you don't increase the stimulus.** I am not talking about time under tension now. I am talking about lifting more weight, doing more reps, or running faster, with each successive workout. It's really as simple as that. Why would anybody work harder for a boss if they weren't going to get more money, more time off, or a better position? Likewise, why would the body change if it doesn't have to? Guess what...it won't!

I am living proof of this. I ran every morning when I was in my early 20's for 3 years. I also lifted religiously. But I did the same weights and the same routines. At the end of that time I looked at pictures and although I felt I was in good shape, I was no bigger, stronger or faster. Why? I had paid my dues, worked out hard, ate right..it wasn't fair! Wrong. It was exactly what it was. My body had become accustomed to a certain speed on my runs, a certain caloric intake, and even the weights I pushed every day.

I finally figured all this out and within 3 months, put on more muscle, ran faster and looked leaner than I had in 3 years. The only thing I did different was write down my weights, cardio times, and food I ate. Then I increased the weights minutely every week, decreased my run times by a few seconds, and manipulated my diet. **I forced my body to change.** Write down all your weights and improve on those every week. If you can't, then it is time to change the exercise, rep range, or body part split. *The body is telling you it has ceased to adapt, so its time to change things up a bit.* If we cease to adapt we will cease to change.

Side note: The power of a log book

I firmly believe you need to document every workout to surpass your previous marks. This is the only way you will continue to make changes and progress. The mind has a funny way of convincing us we are working hard when we are not. If you document everything, you will know exactly what you have to accomplish the next week. Its right there in front of you. That is a powerful motivator, knowing you got 8 ½ reps last week and knowing you have to get 9 this week. It really works. It is also impossible to get stronger forever and by taking notes, you will know when to change and how much you have progressed. Once again, if you find you are not progressing on a certain lift, then it's time to change. It can be as simple as the width of your grip or going to a different exercise completely This will allow for a new stimulus. Once you stop progressing, make a change, or your body transformation will stop.

Blood Flow and Occlusion:

You must increase occlusion and blood flow to your muscles with specific training protocols.
These are vital components to making gains and initiating repair. The more blood flow through the muscle, the more nutrients and growth factors will contribute to your gains. There has been much talk recently about increasing the capillary beds of muscles through increased blood flow. This will essentially increase the muscles growth potential and repair ability. By sustaining a pump through higher reps and increased tension times, you will feel what many have referred to as "the pump." A recent Japanese study also spoke about how vital **occlusion** is to making gains. Whenever you contract a muscle, specifically with contraction-type exercises, you inhibit blood flow from getting there. Once the set is terminated, a massive amount of blood flows into the muscle, and that is when is seems to benefit the most. Hence, blood flow and occlusion work in tandem.

This study pointed out that the massive influx of blood (blood flow), following the lack of it (occlusion), seemed to increase strength and initiate grow factors in the tissue. Plus, the more blood flowing though your muscles, the more BCAA, creatine, glutamine and other workout supplements you consume will follow. Blood flow/occlusion can best be accomplished with exercises that enhance the contraction aspect of a muscle such as concentration curls, leg extensions, tricep pushdowns, kickbacks, and lateral raises. Holding each contraction for one second before the next rep makes them more effective, as well as adding drop sets, super sets, and x-reps.

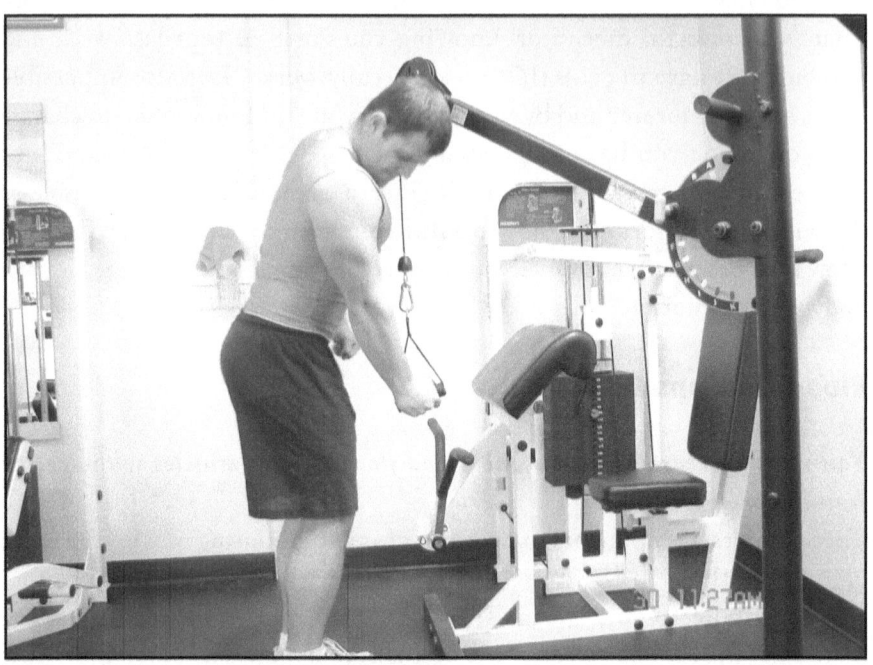

Exercises that enhance contraction of the muscle, in this case the triceps, can greatly enhance occlusion and subsequent blood flow.

Focus on the Negative:

You must focus on controlling the weight throughout the entire repetition. This principle is so often over looked it funny. Study after study have shown that the negative, or eccentric part of the lift, is far superior to the lifting, or concentric aspect. This simply means you should focus on controlling the weight all the way down on every rep. Many individuals find themselves trying to get all ten reps of their set, and drop the weight after each one to gain momentum for the next. Well, this may look good on paper as you'll document getting those reps, but it is killing your gains. You must treat the negative as importantly as the positive. The negative produces more muscle and strength gains than the positive. Without it, you are severely derailing your gains. Every effective program should focus on the negative.

Remember how we talked about the vital importance of time under tension? Well, what happens when you drop the weight or throw it? You lose tension. It may only be for a brief time but it is still lost. Now, when we refer to the positive, or **concentric** part of the lift, we are talking about lifting the weight or contracting the muscle. When we discuss the **negative, or eccentric part of the lift,** we are referring to lowering the weight or elongating the muscle. There is *far more stress on a muscle during the negative portion of the lift than the positive.* This results in more strength and muscle growth. You are far better off to control the negative than to drop the weight in hopes you may gain another rep.

In a recent study, muscles in two groups of athletes were compared after a training session. One group did only concentric lifts and the other was limited to eccentric, or the negative aspect of the lift. After comparing concentric lifts (contraction) vs. eccentric (the negative), far more muscle damage was seen in the eccentric group. This tells us that if you want to build the most muscle, you must put as much, if not more emphasis on the negative as you do the positive. I noticed amazing changes when I started to do this and my strength went through the roof, not to mention severely reducing injuries.

As an example, if it takes me 2 seconds to do a barbell curl, I would want to take a minimum of 2 seconds to lower with control and focus. Often at the end of my sets, I'll have my partner help pull the weight up for me, with as little help as possible. I then lower the weight very slowly and controlled. These are called **forced reps.** Sometimes I'll perform a **static hold** in which I hold the weight in one place towards the bottom of the lift as long as I possibly can. A **pure negative set** is when you use a weight that in no way could be lifted by yourself. Your partner, who obviously must be present, will aid in lifting the weight, and you must lower it as slowly as you can. An example would be placing 50 pounds more than your maximum bench press on the bar and then have your partner help you raise it. Then you lower it in a very slow and controlled manner.

Although I believe controlling the negative is essential on all lifts, <u>*static holds, forced reps, and pure negative sets are best used only occasionally*</u>. These advanced techniques are brutal but should only be used now and then to initiate maximum growth.

Going to slow on the negative can be counterproductive and lead to over-training when used to often. So, all I am advocating is to control the weight, feeling the muscle on the way down as well as on the way up. This not only increases the tension time, but is crucial to building quality muscle. Variation in the speed of the negative is also important and should be changed often. One week take 2 seconds to lower the weight, and maybe 4 seconds the following week. Variability again is key. While you can alter the length of time you perform a negative, again, the most important thing is to control the weight. The rest will fall into place.

Stretch:

You must progressively overload the muscle in the stretch position while lifting; and perform a prolonged stretch of each muscle worked after training.

Progressively overloading the muscle in the stretch position while lifting is crucial to initiate growth. Likewise, stretching the muscle trained vigorously following your lifting session greatly increases the growth and repair process. I never used to stretch or use that many lifts in which the stretch component was emphasized. But since I started, my recovery time has been cut in half and my muscles growth has shot up. It is a very simple aspect of your training protocol that can make a dramatic difference.

The muscles stretch response has just recently been talked about more and more in the fitness and bodybuilding world. A recent study showed that by increasing the resistance in the stretch position of a muscle, over the course of time, yielded a 300% increase in muscle size. That is not a typo! Now, this study was first of all performed on a bird and percentages can be misleading. What we need to take from this study though is that muscle hypertrophy (growth) is **significantly** increased when resistance is applied in the elongated or stretch position. By progressively overloading the muscle in the stretch position, as they did in the study mentioned above, the growth response was greatly accelerated. This essentially means we should increase the resistance with each workout when performing flyes, overhead extensions, pullovers, and incline curls, just to name a few.

We must however use caution and common sense to not overextend the joint or muscle, as this will eventually lead to injury. The stretch position puts the muscle in a vulnerable position so be careful. As long as you warm up properly and use slow, controlled movements with perfect form, you will be fine. Feel the muscle stretch, hold it, and then push back up while keeping constant tension on the muscle. You don't know what sore is until you really work the stretch position, but the results are well worth it. If you don't feel comfortable increasing the weight anymore, then increase the time it takes to lower it. This again is another way to progressively increase resistance by not adding any more physical weight to the lift.

Now, what about after the lift? Again, we must stretch the muscle. In this case we are performing a "static" hold or a basic stretch such as when you lean away from a wall, grab an overhead bar, etc, and stretch the specific muscle. I am not talking about a "walk in the park conversation holding" stretch. The stretch I am talking about must be "uncomfortable." What you are trying to do is stretch the fascia, which is the muscle covering, to allow more room for the muscle to grow. Some studies and many physiologists theorize that the reason many muscles don't grow is because the fascia is inhibiting the growth. So, by completing a deep, uncomfortable stretch (it really burns!), you will not only induce growth but recover much faster.

In summary, after you train the muscle using a stretch exercise, be it biceps, legs, chest or shoulders, it doesn't matter...stretch!! Hold it for 30-60 seconds, it won't be fun and only do it once or twice per workout, definitely **not after every lift**. I usually don't use weights to stretch but you can for certain muscles. An example would be holding dumbbells still in the stretch position following flyes. In any case, I like to perform one stretch *immediately* after the last set for a given body part, preferably the exercise in which I emphasize the stretch component. No more than that. Once again, the purpose is to stretch the fascia to allow more growth and aid in recovery. Don't hurt yourself and go too far. Just use common sense and slowly stretch until you feel the muscle burn. Hold it there for

30-60 seconds and then gently relax. Progressively overloading the stretch position while lifting, and using extreme stretches after your sessions are underutilized techniques, but ones that truly work.

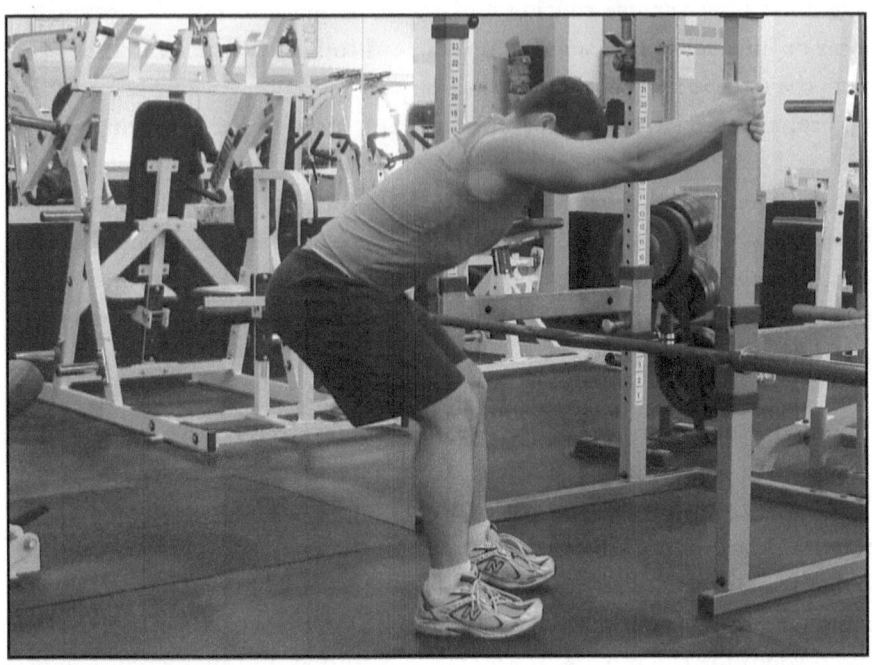

Following your last exercise with a prolonged stretch, in this case the lats, can greatly enhance recovery and growth.

Variability:

You must change your training schemes often to continue making gains. Variability in your training scheme is key. The body is the finest machine you will ever own and eventually will adapt to any training system you embark upon. While gains may come quickly in the beginning, they won't go on forever unless you consistently change the stimulus. Once your body adapts to a specific workout, and you plateau, you must initiate a change. I have found that changing my training protocol, at a minimum every 6 weeks, to be most efficient. Not only does this continue to keep the body guessing, but it prevents you from losing your intensity. If you do the same thing in life, over and over again, how can you maintain the same drive?

Variability in exercises, rep speeds, and days of the week are just a few examples of how you can include variability into your training programs. It can be as simple as switching to a different exercise or alternating which body parts are trained on specific days. Force the body to change by never allowing it to adapt. This will ensure that you will continue to gain.

Time off

You must take time off to regroup, mentally and physically.
There is a time when you must ease up and regroup. Nobody can get stronger and faster forever, no matter how much we change the stimulus. Therefore, I recommend taking a week off, or training very lightly ever 9-12 weeks. This will give you a much-needed rest and re-motivate you to make even greater gains. In due time, no matter how fast or long you have progressed, you will find that the progress plateaus. Then you may find your motivation and drive start to decline, or nagging injuries becoming more prevalent. These are all signs to ease up and take time off. I'll be honest and say that I never just sit around the house and do nothing. I will usually jog casually, stretch, lift without pushing it, play pick-up football games, or go for a bike ride. I just crank the intensity way down and regroup. The brain needs a break just as much as the muscles and joints.

If there is one thing I have learned through the years, **listen to your body.** If you feel ill or your knees and shoulders hurt, back off. More individuals have sustained serious injuries because they failed to shift into a lower gear when the early signs of over training kicked in. Train hard, listen to your body, and know when its time to cut back. You will see greater gains by implementing these actions into your life.

Summary of the Eight Principles Of Resistance Training

1. **High Intensity-**train hard and with a purpose.

2. **Time Under Tension-**try to keep tension on the muscle for at least 30 seconds with controlled reps and/or extended set techniques. The CNS will often quit long before the muscle is stimulated enough to initiate maximum growth. Use drop sets, supersets, x reps/partials, or negatives

to get past this roadblock. High volume, or a large number of sets, is also an option. Both should never be used together though as I believe you can achieve as much growth, with less injury, using low volume and advanced-extended set techniques. See what works for you though. While low reps are required every few weeks to maximize testosterone production and increase CNS output, muscle hypertrophy occurs most often with increased tension times and moderate rep ranges (8-12).

3. **Progressive Overload**-try to improve on each lift at every workout. You can accomplish this by lifting more weight, doing the same amount of reps in less time, etc. Always work to get better and keep a logbook. You must force the body to change. Once you fail to progress, its time to change the lift and/or workout.

4. **Blood Flow and Occulsion**: try to increase the amount of blood flow to a muscle while lifting to increase capillary beds and nutrient influx. This can be accomplished with occlusion of the muscle through higher reps or contraction type exercises. A subsequent increase in blood flow will usually follow the set. Contracted exercises best accomplish this such as concentration curls, cable cross-overs, tricep pushdowns, kick-backs, rows, leg extensions, and lateral raises. Incorporating x-reps, drop sets, and super sets with these lifts can dramatically make them more effective.

5. **Focus on the Negative**-the muscle is most stimulated to grow through the eccentric, or negative aspect of the lift. Don't just focus on lifting the weight, you must control the range of motion throughout the entire rep.

6. **Stretch**- make sure at least one exercise for each body part utilizes the stretch position and try to make progress each week. Also, stretch for 30-60 seconds after the last exercise for each muscle group. You will grow and recover much faster using these techniques.

7. **Variability**-you must change your workouts schemes often to prevent plateaus. At a minimum, changes should occur every 6 weeks. I prefer to change every week, which I'll explain more later. If you are still

gaining each workout, by all means keep going. Most however start to fatigue mentally or physically after 6 weeks, and a change is needed.

8. **Time Off**-every 9-12 weeks take a complete week off or turn the intensity way down. No high intensity techniques or going to failure. The CNS and body must regroup or you will begin to succumb to over training.

Commonly Asked Questions

What exercises should I focus on?

Now that we have covered the principles to key on while training, we should discuss more specific exercise techniques. In this section I will not so much discuss exercises, but rather the range of motions I think are most beneficial. In so doing, the specific exercises will fall into place. There are three aspects of a muscles range of motion that should be incorporated into each workout. These include a *mid range, stretch, and contraction* movement for the specific body part being trained. Steve Holman at Iron Man magazine, the inventor of Positions of Flexion (POF), does a great job of describing these in his book, *Train, Eat, Grow: Position- of- Flexion Muscle- Training Manual*, which I urge you all to look into.

Midrange movements include lifts such as presses, squats, barbell curls, skull crushers and dead lifts. These lifts generate maximum force and quickly stimulate the high threshold motor units. **Stretch** position movements include incline curls, flyes, pullovers, and overhead extensions. When it comes to these, I use caution and really work on stretching the muscle before contracting again. Perform each stretch movement slowly and with focus, as poor form on these lifts can lead to injury. **Contraction** movements would include concentration curls, cable crossovers, pushdowns, and lateral raises to name a few. Once again, these are ideal to increase TUT and maximize blood flow/occlusion.

Many overlook exactly what range of motion they are doing with a particular lift, but I believe them to be an important piece to the muscle-building puzzle. A trainee should make sure all three positions are stimulated during their workout for the specific muscle being trained. Incorporating the eight principles into mid-range, stretch, and contraction movements can lead to very impressive gains. Although you can do all of these movements with machines or cables, I tend to do mid range movements with compound lifts and use machines to work the stretch and contraction aspects. The reason I like compound lifts is that they allow for more muscle fiber recruitment and heavier weights. The cables and machines allow for more control and isolation. As a general rule, the lower the rep range, the more you should cater towards compound lifts as they have the greatest propensity to build muscle. All in all, there are no rules and one should make sure to use variety in their lifting schemes.

How often should I train?

This question is at the forefront of any workout program and is often the most confusing. The answer really relates to how well you recover and how intense your workouts are. I promise you, nothing is worse than putting your body into an over trained state. All you are trying to do is stimulate the muscle enough to initiate a positive change. Nothing more. If you go above and beyond that, the results will be negative.

Think of it this way. You go out on a hot, sunny day and spend 2 hours in the sun. The next day you realize you have a perfect tan. The next week, you really want a darker tan and spend 4 hours in the sun. The day after you have a terrible sunburn and it takes a couple weeks to recover before you dare go out there again. Weight training is no different. Causing just enough damage on a consistent basis will yield the best results. Too little and it does nothing, too much, and you are in an over trained state. It truly is a fine line. So, here is the way I approach most training programs.

Train each body part no more than once every 72 hours and no less than once per week. I prefer to train each muscle once per week.

Studies have shown that training legs more than once per week can be counter productive. They are your largest muscle group and take a tremendous toll on your body, not only to train, but in recovery as well. Upper body muscles can be trained every 72 hours, but I have found once per week to be ideal for a natural athlete. Now, there are individuals who train legs twice and chest three times per week but this is not the norm. More and more magazines tout such programs, but for the natural athlete, it often is too much. In time, individuals on these frequent, high volume workouts become injured or so fatigued they can't work hard enough to cause positive changes or even recover.

There are individuals though that benefit from these multiple workouts but I don't recommend starting there. Should you find that you aren't progressing on once a week workouts, then you can slowly add another session. If you go this route though, you should severely reduce the number of sets in your workout. In this case you must train intensely but with a lower volume set-up. This way you will recover faster and thus get by with more frequent workouts.

I do periodically train upper body parts every 4-5 days but within 4-5 weeks find that I grow tired, irritable, and lose my drive. If I wait 7 days, I am fired up and ready to go again. For some, like myself, this frequency works well. I train extremely hard though and if I do this too often (more than once per week), will actually put myself in a state of over training. Some that train once per week will notice that they get stronger each week but their gains in muscle size are often lacking. This is simply because the muscles often are repaired and ready to be trained again a few days before the CNS.
We must remember that the CNS is one of the main reasons our muscles essentially stop firing, even though they have a lot more in them. Therefore, for a percentage of the population, I feel more success is found in training all upper body muscles once every 4-5 days. The only way to know is to see how intense your workouts are, how fast you recover, how much sleep you get, how sound your diet is, etc. As you can see, it changes from person to person. *In summary, I suggest training each body part with intense workouts once per week and see how you recover.* Remember that we grow after the workout, not during, and our main goal is to stimulate the fibers to adapt and grow later. Any more than that will yield negative results. We always think that more is better, and for natural athletes, that can often be the furthest thing from the truth.

Should I use high volume or low volume?

Now, as mentioned before, some trainees only have confidence and see gains with high volume training. I think if you incorporate what we talked about earlier, you can cut your work sets way down. If not, you must reduce your frequency if you train with high volume. Again, I have tried high volume workouts with sets approaching 20-25 per body part but never understood how you could give everything you had for 20 sets? If I did, I found that I either sustained an injury or grew sick of the gym. If you train hard you can get the job done in 6-12 sets per body part.

Here's the catch though. *If you reduce the volume you must increase the intensity.* Period! Don't think that just because you cut your sets way down means it will be easier. In fact, you may wish you did 20 sets at half the intensity these programs call for. By training this way, you can hit body parts more intensely and thus stimulate more growth. If you eat poorly or don't get enough sleep, it may be too much, no matter what program you follow. If you do train with a high volume program, you should not incorporate extended set techniques and limit your sets to failure. High volume is a valid way to overcome CNS failure, but I believe you can achieve similar results with low volume and advanced-extended set techniques such as drop sets, forced reps, super sets, x-reps, and negatives. Plus, you can do it in half the time.

Which rep range should I focus on?

All of them! I am serious when I say that to maximize muscle growth all fibers must be stimulated, although not necessarily in the same workout. It is important to realize that training with drop sets, partials, and other advanced techniques is beneficial most of the time, but it can't be a constant. In fact, if you trained with these techniques 100% of the time, you are sure to succumb to over training, as well as miss out on other areas of growth. Not to mention the boredom and lack of variety a workout like this would entail.

In saying that, I urge all of you to look into the teachings of Eric Broser. Mr. Broser is one of the finest trainers in the country and 100% natural. I have had the privilege of working with him personally and to say his teachings and programs are effective would be a gross understatement. His programs focus around a principle he invented called Power-Rep Range-Shock (P/RR/S). Mr. Broser essentially divides each week into one of the above techniques and thus initiates variety into his workouts, as well as his mental fortitude. It is no surprise that this works as we already covered variation as being one of the principles to consistent gains.

With the P/RR/S system, the **power** week is performed with all exercises done in the 4-6 rep range. Compound lifts are emphasized and no partials, drop sets, or other advanced techniques should be incorporated. The negative should be slow and controlled. A few forced reps can be thrown in there on the last set for each body part but that's it! Time under tension is not as long as the other weeks but our goal here is to tap into the high threshold fibers immediately and quickly stimulate more motor units. This often shocks the CNS, builds strength quickly, and increases testosterone production. Rest periods are 2-4 minutes between sets. It is almost a down-regulated week as there will be little lactic acid accumulation. Don't worry though, the deep muscle soreness that follows will remind you it was anything but an easy week!

The **rep range** week follows and usually prescribes three different exercises and rep ranges. The first is 3-4 sets of 7-9 reps, the second 2-3 sets of 10-12, and the third 2-3 sets of 13-20 reps. This truly fatigues and stimulates all the fiber types and focuses most of the reps in the hypertrophy or growth zone. If you are focused and control the negative, the time under tension is adequate and muscle hypertrophy is greatly increased. Although the final reps are higher, they are still enhancing growth. Your fast twitch muscle fibers are already fatigued from the previous sets, which makes tapping into the last few fibers much easier. With higher reps, occlusion and increased blood flow also become important components to growth.

This is in contrast to those who seek to get leaner or "tone" up, and do all their exercises in the 20-rep range with light weights. These individuals are doing the exact opposite of what they should be doing, and are merely building up their endurance or slow twitch fibers. Worse, they are not "forcing" the body to preserve or create new muscle tissue. **Adding more**

muscle will do nothing but increase our metabolism and make us more toned. That is the mistake many make, thinking the use of high reps will build definition. The only thing that will do, again, is build endurance in the slow twitch fibers and slow muscle growth. If you train with heavier weights though, reach positive failure and fatigue the muscle, *higher reps that follow will then force the muscle to call upon even more fibers,* not to mention increasing blood flow and occlusion. The Rep Range week is a perfect example of how one can and should use higher reps to initiate growth.

The final week is **shock** week. This is where you completely destroy the muscles with advanced techniques such as x-reps, drop sets, multi-rep rest pause training and forced reps. The number of sets is reduced, but as we have talked about, the more intense the stimulation, the less volume is needed. I add partials or x-reps to all my lifts during shock week and often finish with a drop set. The number of exercises and sets must be personalized per individual but I often only do four supersets and one drop set per body part. Believe me, you'll be thankful shock week only occurs once every three weeks!

Why it Works

This program is great in many ways. Straight power weeks allow for a downgrade in training without you even knowing it. It taxes the CNS greatly and while you'll notice the pump isn't as pronounced, the CNS is stimulated to handle heavier weights and therefore activate more motor units. A trainee's strength will shoot through the roof with these power workouts. This isn't bad though as within a few days you'll start pounding the muscles during rep range week. This week adds new stimuli by increasing TUT and decreasing rest periods. Then shock week arrives and the protocol changes again! This time you are greatly increasing blood flow, occlusion, and endurance. Rest periods are minimal and the sets are prolonged. This means all fibers are stimulated, strength *and* endurance, as well as enhancing lactic acid production. Find what works best for you but remember, variation is key and this program hits all eight principles right on the head. I'll outline my personal P/RR/S program at the end of this chapter and for more information go to www.prrstraining.com.

Which muscles do I train on each day?

As far as which muscles to pair up, once again in depends on many factors. I believe in training with the notion that there are supporting muscle groups that are indirectly worked each session. Simply put, if you train chest, you are hitting the triceps and shoulders as well, albeit indirectly. If you are training mid-back and lats, you are hitting the biceps. So, the last thing you would want to do is hit back hard on Monday and then follow that up with biceps on Tuesday. You are better off to train them on the same day or at least 72 hours apart.

I actually find it advantageous to hit chest individually with shoulders and/or triceps in separate workouts. Chest exercises thoroughly hit my shoulders and triceps, and therefore work them indirectly. In separating my shoulder and chest workouts, I make sure that they are at least three days apart as to not over train the shoulder joint. If you can't separate them by at least 3 days, it is again better to train them on the same day. The same goes for back and biceps, or hamstrings and quadriceps. Once again, you may find incorporating chest, triceps and shoulders works great for you, so by all means find the set up that works best and go with it.

Another great method, and my preference, is to work agonist and antagonist muscle groups in the same workout. This means if I do chest, I follow that up with back or biceps in the same session. If I do quadriceps, I follow that with hamstring work. This provides a tremendous pump and allows you to work the entire muscle with maximum effort. If you did back on Monday, and biceps on Tuesday, the bicep workout would suffer as you have already fatigued them during back work the day before. The same goes for following a chest workout with triceps.

Yet another technique is the push/pull set-up. This entails hitting "push" muscles on the same day such as chest/triceps/shoulders and "pull" on another day such as back and biceps. Once again, there are no rules, but I have found the greatest gains and least amount of injury by pairing agonist/antagonist or push/pull body parts into the same workout. I have listed a few of my favorite set-ups below.

Example Pairings (Agonist/Antagonist): M/W/F

1. Chest/Back

2. Quadriceps/Hamstrings/Calves

3. Biceps/Triceps/Shoulders

Example Pairings (Push/Pull): M/W/F

1. Chest/Triceps/Shoulders...Push muscles get worked together

2. Quadriceps/Hamstrings/Calves

3. Back/Biceps...Pull muscles get worked together.

Example 4 day split: M/T/OFF/TR/F

1. Chest/Biceps

2. Quadriceps/Hamstrings/Calves

3. OFF

4. Back

5. Triceps/Shoulders

I Never Follow this Split:

1. Chest on Monday

2. Triceps/Shoulders on Tuesday (Chest soreness will limit tricep/shoulder lifts and inhibit chest recovery)

3. Biceps on Wednesday

4. Back on Thursday (Bicep soreness will limit back strength and inhibit bicep recovery)

5. Legs on Friday

Keep these things in mind when setting up your program!

Free Weights vs. Machines

I am writing this section simply because it is such a confusing area for many athletes. Every magazine you pick up, every book you read, has its opinions and many are valid. The one myth I want to dispel though is that machines are inferior to free weights. Machines have their time and place, just like free weights do. I firmly believe that lifting with free weights are extremely important to gain mass, increase strength, work the stabilizer muscles, and push yourself to the limit. Machines allow me to focus less on stabilizing the weight and more on directly stimulating the muscle I want. These statements point to the simple fact that <u>**one should incorporate both into their workouts.**</u>

In fact, the toughest workouts I have completed have had equal representation from both free weights and machines. Many believe they will never be able to attain a great physique because they only have access to a few machines in their basement or gym. It is far more important to focus on the eight principles we discussed earlier than the quality of your gym.
I like to use machines as finishing movements and as part of supersets. An example would be lat pulldowns after chins and cable curls after dumbbell or barbell curls. With free weights, you have the ability to move more weight and better develop the stabilizer muscles that are part of all compound movements. Machines on the other hand allow for a more controlled lift and therefore can allow you to better maintain the "time under tension" we talked about earlier. Using both free weights and machines are important, and both should be used to construct the ideal program.

Form

I can't tell you how many people, including myself at one time, lifted with poor form just to get that extra weight and say they did it. This technique, or lack thereof, does nothing but invite injury and will never help you in the long run. You should always mix your lifts up and become an expert at all of them. Some may not be able to squat, but do great on a leg press. Some may hate barbell curls but get tremendous gains off of dumbbell curls. <u>**Don't ever let anyone lead you down the wrong path if you know its not good for you.**</u> In time you will find the best lifts and the ones you feel comfortable doing. Care must be taken though to prevent you from becoming lazy and unwilling to try new techniques and programs. Learn the correct form and try to become an expert at all lifts. In time, you will see greater muscular gains than the guy who is using more momentum than muscle to get those last few reps.

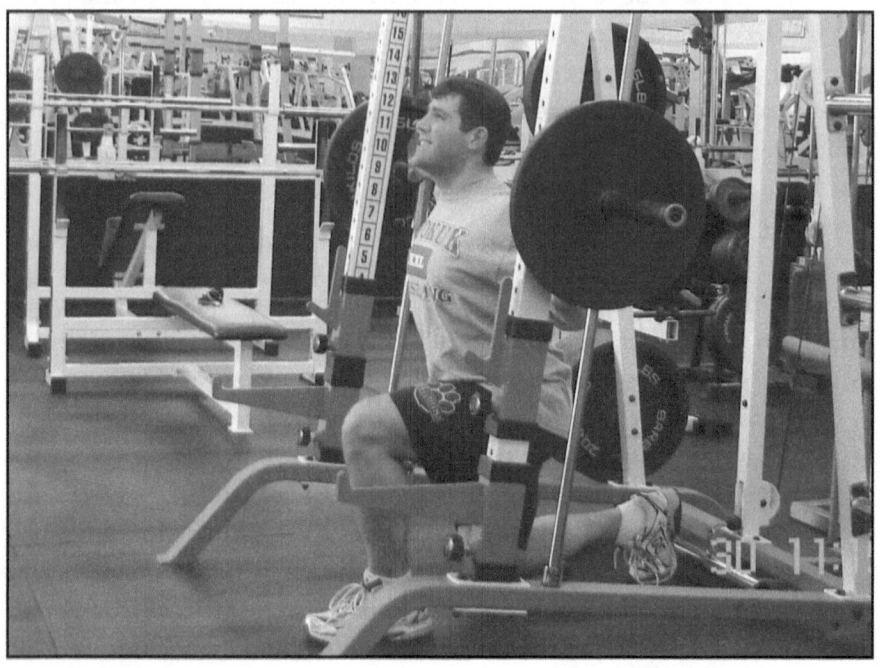

No matter which lifts you decide to incorporate into your training programs, practice good form and the gains are sure to follow.

Is Cheating Ever Allowed?

There are times when you can cheat to get that last rep, *but they should be used with caution, only on certain lifts, and with experienced lifters only.* Sometimes using a little swing to aid in the last rep of a dumbbell curl, or your legs to help get the last upright row can really torch those last few fibers needed for growth. On the other hand, cheating on dead lifts or squats is nothing but ignorant and can lead to a lifetime of back pain. As a general rule, always practice good form and the gains will come in good time.

As you can see, the possible workout schemes are endless. I promise, if I showed you one scheme, another would be in the next magazine or book you read, and the confusion starts all over. I will detail the workouts I use at the end of this book, but realize that you can develop the ideal program yourself. There is no "perfect" program, just perfect for you! Practice the eight principles and keep making steady progress, the rewards will be well worth it.

Lets summarize the keys to building a solid program.

My preferences are as follows:

- Train each body part once per week and only then decide whether you need to increase the frequency.
- Never train with weights more than 4 days per week and never more than two days in a row.
- Generally use 8-12 sets for shoulders/chest/back/legs and 6 sets for biceps, triceps and calves.
- Separate your workouts into different repetition protocols.
- I prefer to train agonist/antagonist or push/pull muscle groups in the same workout but find what best works for you.
- Incorporate the eight principles discussed no matter what program you follow.

The eight principles and various techniques we have just discussed, if followed, will allow you to reach your goals. They truly are part of every successful training protocol I have come across. As you read more magazines and books, you will notice these philosophies and principles scattered among the hundreds of programs printed every year. Although I find Eric Broser's P/RR/S programs to be one of the best, I urge all of you to create your ideal program, one you believe in, and one that is designed to achieve your goals. Focus on the eight principles, decide on the lifts you have the most confidence in, the days of the week in which you train, and the body part splits you will follow. Above all, know what you are trying to achieve, and be specific in your goals. The rest will fall into place.

Chapter 7

CARDIOVASCULAR AND WEIGHT TRAINING TO MAXIMIZE FAT LOSS

Cardiovascular Training to Maximize Fat Loss

Cardiovascular training is vital to attain the physique you desire. It is a must. I firmly believe that diet is 75% of what we look like, but without cardiovascular training, the puzzle is incomplete, and you will never attain the lean look you desire. Even if you are reading this book with the soul interest in gaining muscle, there will come a time when you will want to reveal the muscle you have developed. Without cardio, you will never accomplish that goal.

Not only is cardio important for overall health, it provides better blood flow to your muscles and prevents excessive fat accumulation. Many argue that they only need to do cardio before summer or a contest. I assure you these individuals have a much harder time getting rid of that extra fat than the individual who performs cardio all year long.

Everybody is different and some will need more cardio than others. In the following section we will discuss what type of cardio is superior, how much you need to do, and what time of day to do it. We will also touch on how the foods you consume can greatly affect how much fat you are able to burn. Cardiovascular training is a vital component in the quest to transform your body.

High Intensity Interval Training (HIIT) vs Low Intensity

There are two theories on cardio: **high intensity vs. low intensity.** High intensity interval training (HIIT) refers to sprints, intervals or cardiovascular exercise in which your heart rate is greatly elevated. The duration is usually less than 20 minutes and fluctuates between high and low speeds. Low intensity is of longer duration with slower speeds, usually referring to any activity over 30 minutes, such as marathons, long jogs or aerobic classes. Which is better? Well, there really isn't a straightforward answer. What I mean is I firmly believe you should do both, and sometimes in the same workout, but we will get to that later.

I love when I read an article, and one lean guy or gal swears they have the answer. Then you read another article, by an author with an equally impressive physique, and they completely contradict what you just solidified as the truth. Well, let me save you all a lot of time and confusion. There is no definitive answer. High intensity has its place, as well as low intensity. We must take into account how healthy your joints are, how much muscle you have, how mentally tough you are, and hell, whether you even like cardio or not.

Aerobic vs Anaerobic

The body is, without a doubt, the most efficient and remarkable machine you will ever own. It knows when you need food, water, and sleep. Likewise, it knows when we can and have to give up fat stores to survive. We as athletes must force and trick the body into giving up its "safety net," or what we call fat reserves. The first thing we all need to do when trying to accomplish a physical change is to ask ourselves, **"What stimulus must I elicit to force my body to change?"** Marathon runners train long grueling miles to force their bodies to become more efficient in fuel consumption and oxygen use. They become so efficient in fact that they often hold onto a "healthy" amount of body fat because the body needs it to support their grueling training. Along the way they often lose a good deal of muscle, which remember, is the most metabolically active tissue in the body.

I have many friends that run marathons and comment on the fact that no matter how far they run they never seem to lose as much body fat as they thought they would. The reason is usually because without a "healthy supply" of body fat to fuel the workout, it becomes difficult to complete 26.2 miles! The body simply becomes more efficient by stripping muscle and making body fat a little more available. Why? Body fat is much easier to use as an energy source than muscle. Also, the less muscle we have the easier it is to hold onto fat stores. So, I think we agree that running 26.2 miles is not necessary to attain the physique we want! Still, long duration cardio has its place, just not in a marathon-type fashion.

Now, lets look at the body of a sprinter. They usually have well defined glutes and legs, larger upper body muscles and less endurance fibers. They primarily use fast twitch fibers as their sprints are explosive and of short duration. Much like lifting weights! In this case, it is almost impossible to access fat that quickly and the body relies more on ATP and glucose. Hence, fat stores need not be present to accomplish the task.

Marathon runners are usually skinnier, have poor muscle definition and amazing endurance. *They are essentially aerobic athletes while sprinters are more anaerobic.* Instead of initially using fat for fuel, sprinters use ATP, and then glycogen stores in the muscles and liver. Glycogen, as you already know, is broken down into glucose, and thus used for fuel via ATP production. The reason the body prefers glucose versus fat, in regards to anaerobic activities, is simply because it is far easier to use as a quick source of energy.

Think of glucose as a money clip where as fat used for fuel needs a couple signatures and an ATM card. *Glucose and ATP are quick energy; fat takes time to tap into.* That is why many people eat sugar cubes and candy bars when they feel tired or weak. **The advantage of lifting weights and doing high intensity cardio is that your metabolism becomes accustomed to processing glucose quickly and efficiently, without storing fat or relying on it for energy.** They are what we refer to as anaerobic exercises. There is no need to store much fat while lifting or performing high intensity cardio because the duration of your activity is short and intense. The body first uses ATP and then glucose that comes from recently eaten carbohydrates or glycogen stores. The benefits don't stop there as anaerobic athletes usually hold onto or gain much more muscle than aerobic athletes, which greatly enhances their ability to burn fat.

I read all the time that you must perform at least 30 minutes of low intensity cardio to burn fat. Tell that to Skip Lacour, a motivational speaker and champion bodybuilder. He does an average of 16-minute <u>high intensity</u> cardio sessions! Now, here's the big difference between HIIT and low intensity cardio: *little fat is burned <u>during</u> high intensity cardio, while low intensity cardio maximizes its fat burning effects <u>during the session</u>.* Now, just because little fat is burned during HIIT, or any anaerobic exercise, doesn't mean it won't happen in the hours that follow! Let me explain.

Good Things Come to Those Who Wait

While high intensity cardio will first tap into glycogen, rather than fat, fat burning will begin to occur, and continue, **in the hours following the workout.** As soon as the available glucose and glycogen is spent, the body must have an energy source to keep going, so it finally taps into its fat reserves. When high intensity cardio is performed, fast and efficiently, fat will be burning all day long. **That's one of the major benefits of high intensity cardio, a much faster metabolism throughout the rest of the day.** Your body is running on all cylinders and burning fat while you are at work, running errands, and even watching TV. The catch is that your workout must be intense and you must push yourself, which takes mental fortitude.

I firmly believe the best way to perform high intensity cardio is to train with intervals. I like to stretch first and then jog a couple of minutes. I then run as fast as can for 1-2 minutes, jog or walk for a minute, and repeat. I do this for 15-20 minutes. You can perform intervals while swimming, biking, walking, or on the elliptical. The key is to take your heart rate to a high level and then back down again. The metabolism gets revved up and in the hours that follow your workout fat loss is your reward. It is brutal but highly effective.

Will Long Duration Cardio Work?

Now, what about long duration? Well, first off, when I say long duration, I mean no more than 1 hour and that is pushing it. If it is marathons you are training for, then the nutrition and training information go beyond this book. We all want to have a lean, healthy look but we don't have to kill ourselves with marathon training sessions. Most marathon and tri-athletes, and these are tremendous athletes we are talking about here, do so for reasons not related to wanting to look ripped or muscular. If marathons are what you want to excel at, go for it! They are extremely difficult and I have the utmost respect for anyone who desires to complete a marathon. However, for the purpose of getting fit, lean, and muscular, hour upon hour of cardiovascular training is not needed.

Why Isn't Longer Better?

When the body starts a cardiovascular event that goes beyond one hour, it realizes that it must become more efficient and begins by ridding itself of some muscle. Why? Well, muscle can be broken down and converted to energy just like fat can. This process provides glucose to the body through a different route called gluconeogenesis. It is just another survival adaptation the body is capable of. So, if your body was forced into performing hours of cardiovascular training, what do you think it would do, use fat or drop muscle? Sure, it will *eventually* tap into fat stores but it will also begin breaking down muscle tissue. Muscle is metabolically demanding and although a much poorer fuel source than fat for long duration aerobic training, it still will be broken down.

Anytime muscle begins to atrophy, it becomes much more difficult to attain a lean, ripped physique. Still, "longer" duration cardio can be an important component to dropping body fat. When I say "longer" duration though, I am referring to 30-60 minutes of cardio, no more. The reason it must be at least 30 minutes is secondary to the time it takes for the body to beginning tapping into fat stores. The low intensity and aerobic nature of this type of cardio requires that the duration be longer, as _the actual fat burning takes place during the session_. Therefore, keeping your times between 30-60 minutes will ensure you still burn fat, while not compromising your muscle tissue.

Do I Need a Heart Rate Monitor for Low Intensity Cardio?

Forget heart rate monitors when doing low intensity cardio. You are at the right level if you have broken a sweat at about 5-6 minutes and can barely hold a conversation throughout the session. The catch is you must perform this for at least 30-45 minutes. Performing long duration cardio at a moderate pace will eventually tap into your fat stores; it just takes longer to get there. The downside is that you won't rev your metabolism up for hours after you are done as you would with high intensity cardio or lifting weights.

So...What's the Best Way?

So, what's the right answer? Well, in my opinion, the answer is both. I usually do a combination session at least twice per week but also alternate days during the week, some high, some low. If I do both in the same session I'll do sprints or intervals to start my sessions, and then finish with a low intensity workout. This is my favorite tactic and that which I believe to be the best. Start with high intensity and finish with low. For example, I prefer to run intervals for the first 10-15 minutes of my cardio session and then slant the treadmill on a steep incline and walk for another 15-30 minutes. The results are amazing. If am outside on a track, I first run sprints and then slowly jog the last 15-30 minutes.

My Favorite Type Of Cardio

Do I have a favorite high and low intensity cardio exercise? You bet! My favorite low intensity cardio technique is walking on a treadmill with an incline. I set the incline at 12 and speed at 3.5 mph. When doing so though *it is important to never hold on*. It takes much less energy to hold on to the treadmill handles and this will reduce the amount of fat you burn. If you find you must hold on then your going to fast. My favorite high intensity cardio workout consists of 400-meter sprints on a track. I often run a 400m sprint (1 lap) and then walk a lap. It absolutely kills me! On average, my

HIIT takes 15-20 minutes, my long duration 45 minutes, and the mixture of the two approximately 30 minutes. Just remember any cardio is better than none and you should find the system that work best for you.

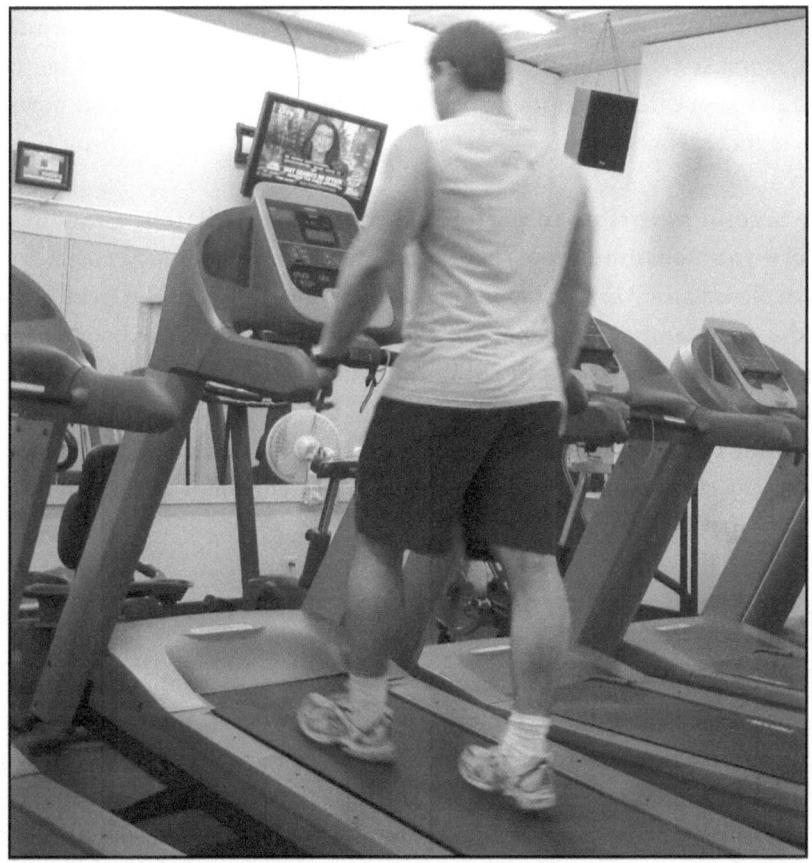

Uphill treadmill walks, while appearing easy, are a challenging and potent fat burning activity. Just remember....Don't Hold On!

What is the Best Time of Day to Do Cardio?

Now, as far as the time of day in which we perform cardio, **there is no better time than first thing in the morning, on an empty stomach.** Again, the reason is that glycogen and glucose levels are at their lowest, which means your body will tap into fat stores immediately. *This trick can burn more fat* *than you ever imagined*. Remember that insulin is released by the pancreas any time we eat. While it is allows us to store food, it's release will also shut down fat loss. It is, after all, a storage hormone. Therefore, if you do cardio first thing in the morning, before you consume any food, especially carbohydrates, insulin will not be released. Instead, glucagon will be the prevalent hormone released and with it comes HSL and other hormones that increase fat metabolism. Add a fat burning supplement to increase the release of catecholamines, such as norepinephrine, and the fat burning effects increase even more!

The second best time to perform cardio is immediately after lifting, before you consume a post workout meal. Once again, glycogen levels are depleted and you will tap into fat stores more quickly. **Not performing cardio on an empty stomach is one of the main reasons cardio programs are not more effective at burning fat.** Many of you think that you could never train in the morning before eating, but you have to if you want to take your physique to the next level. In fact, many fitness professionals do a morning session and another immediately after weight raining to double the fat burning effect.

Cardio Should Follow Weight Training

Why not do cardio first and then lift? Well, you want as much glycogen in your muscles as possible to fuel your weight training sessions. After lifting, the reduced glycogen stores will make it easier to tap into fat during your cardio session. Glycogen will be nearly depleted, and once that occurs, fat is next to be metabolized. Studies have also found a greater amount of fat burning hormones, just as GH and IGF-1, are produced if you do your weight training session before cardio. I personally have found my strength is greatly reduced if I do cardio first, and therefore try to separate the two events as far as possible. One option is to do cardio first thing in the morning and then return after work to lift. A second option, and one that most prefer, is to perform your cardio in the morning on days you don't train with weights, and immediately after on days that you do.

That way you only have to make one trip to the gym. No matter when you perform cardio though, **it is essential to consume 5-10 g of BCAA and**

glutamine before cardio to inhibit muscle loss. This means a drink before your morning session or immediately following lifting weights. This will not inhibit fat loss, give you a sensation of consuming food, and protect your hard earned muscle. I feel one should increase the amount to 20 g of BCAA and 10 g of glutamine if your cardio takes place after lifting. This is in addition to your shakes consumed while training. Again, this will initiate the repair process right after lifting and protect you from burning muscle and becoming catabolic.

If you consume your normal post workout drink immediately after lifting and before cardio, it will blunt fat burning secondary to the insulin spike. Consuming BCAA and glutamine before performing cardio, then consuming your normal post-workout drink will give you all the benefits and still allow you to burn fat. Less BCAA and glutamine is needed in the morning as you haven't been training and are merely trying to stave off muscle loss. No doubt about it, BCAA and glutamine are essential.

Performing a mixture of high and low intensity cardio, first thing in the morning or after lifting, can take your physique to new levels. If you prefer high intensity or low intensity, by all means perform that which suits you best. Any cardio is better than none! Just remember, the slower you go, the longer your session must be. Now, lets talk about how we can manipulate our weight training workouts to burn more fat.

Weight Training Protocols for Maximum Fat Loss

Many factors go into fat loss, with diet and cardio being the major players. Now, lets take it a step further and expand on what we have already talked about. There are ways to train that will maximize hormone production and increase fat loss. It isn't so much the workout, but how you go about it that is important when training to lose body fat.

Reduce Rest Periods to Increase Fat Loss

The first technique and one that is often thought to be used, but rarely is, deals with rest periods. <u>**If you really want to increase your metabolism and accelerate fat loss, you must decrease the time in takes you to go**</u>

from set to set. Now, I want to make a point in regards to the type of training you will be doing with reduced rest between sets. All programs will work, including the ones I will outline at the end of this book. By just reducing your rest periods and training with maximum intensity, you can burn more fat. When it comes to weight training with fat loss as my primary goal, I rarely rest more than 1 minute between sets. This ensures I keep my metabolism elevated, which greatly aids the loss of body fat.

Like I said, in regards to lifting, there is no special program. It is more about **principles**, techniques you can use on any program to make it more effective. Likewise, there is no specific amount of rest that will always work. One minute rest periods between sets is a good place to start if growth hormone production is our primary goal. GH, as you remember from our previous section on hormones, is a major fat catalyst. Sometimes I train with 30 seconds of rest between sets, and other times I wait 90 seconds. I never go more than 2 minutes though unless I am training for maximize strength, such as during power week of the P/RR/S program. So now you're thinking, "I get it, reduce and vary my rest periods, this increases metabolism and intensity!" Correct, but there is another reason few know about, and that reason is lactic acid.

Lactic Acid

Lactic acid, as we touched on earlier in this book, is responsible for the "burn" I know we have all felt at one point or another. Similarly, lactic acid production, through intense training, is one of the main proponents of growth hormone. The natural production of growth hormone initiates the use of fat for fuel and increases our metabolism for hours after our workout is complete. By reducing the rest periods between sets, we can increase lactic acid and maximize the production of GH; thus fat burning increases. Every time you lift a weight, you are using glycogen as fuel (remember, that which is stored in our muscles from glucose). As we are burning glycogen, lactic acid is produced as a by- product, and initiates the burn we have all come to know so well. Well, if lactic acid means we are burning up glycogen, that means eventually we will start burning fat! With intense training and reduced rest periods, you will cause the body to become a hormone producing-fat burning machine!

Now, if you can perform this type of workout with just enough fuel to keep you going, which keeps insulin levels low, the body will tap into fat stores more readily. Remember, having low glycogen and insulin levels promotes fat loss. Combine that with cardio and intense workouts, and you will see results like never before. Many of us feel that we couldn't possibly work out at that level of intensity without some food. The truth however remains that you will burn the most fat, and initiate the most growth hormone production, with a very low amount of insulin in your blood. So, the key is to take in just enough carbohydrates and protein to get you through the workout.

I have found that if I consume 10-20 g of BCAA and 5-10 g of glutamine in a drink mix that I can push right through a workout and keep insulin stable. While we discussed earlier the advantage of adding Gatorade powder to your workout drink mix, it should be excluded in this case if fat loss is our primary goal. The BCAA and glutamine will keep cortisol blunted and muscle loss at a minimum. Again, Scivation makes an awesome product called X-Tend that is a BCAA/ glutamine mix. I add 6 scoops to a shaker bottle and sip it the entire workout. It tastes great. Another good glutamine/ BCAA mix is made by Xtreme formulations and is called ICE.

Rep Ranges for Maximum Fat Loss

The last thing I'll comment on when weight training to maximize fat loss is the reps schemes themselves. The most common thing you hear in gyms is the theory that you should lift in the high rep range when trying to get ripped, and low rep range when trying to get big. Well, ___nothing could be further from the truth___. The type of high reps those trying to get ripped often propose is 3 sets of 20 reps, stopping often at that number.

For one thing, why are we always talking about 3 sets? It seems to be an arbitrary number to me. There is nothing special about it. Also, why stop at 20 reps, why not 18 or 22? **You see, the key is to go to maximum muscle failure.** Your goal might be 20, but if you hit 17 or 18 and fail at 100% effort, then you have stimulated that muscle properly. We are trying to create the leanest, most muscular physique we can, and the easiest way to do that is through muscle gains and preservation. To do that, we need to follow the techniques as outlined in the previous sections and lift to failure with challenging weights. Whether it be 6 or 20 reps-perform them with intensity and push to failure. This will ensure we hold onto as much muscle as possible while we lose body fat. The more muscle we have, the faster our metabolism, and the more fat we'll burn.

While the P/RR/S protocol I follow varies rep ranges from 4-20, studies again have shown the **greatest muscle growth occurs in the 8-12 rep range**. We must force the body to hold onto muscle while we strip away body fat. If you lift with high reps and stop short of failure, you will merely increase the endurance component of the muscle and not necessarily stimulate it to grow. No matter the goal I am after, getting bigger or leaner, I still lift hard and with weights that push me to failure. Again, diet and cardio are the big keys to getting leaner, with specific lifting programs being the least important. *In fact, my workouts stay the same whether my goal is to get bigger or leaner-I just reduce my rest periods and alter my diet.*

Should you design your own program though, please refrain from the concept that you need extremely high reps to get leaner. Also, **don't believe that lifting isn't essential if all you really care about is losing body fat.** You must lift to increase metabolism, strip body fat, and preserve muscle. This goes for either sex. I promise, set your nutrition protocol towards getting leaner, perform cardio, lift hard, and the only side effect will be a lean, toned physique.

ABS

I am adding this at the end of the fat loss section for one reason: it fits! No other body part screams "in- shape" more than the abdominals. If you have a guy with huge arms and a large stomach, he won't be regarded nearly as "in-shape" as the skinny guy with a six-pack. Sad but true. I promise, you can do all the crunches, ab-isolations, and 6-minute fixes you want, but it won't matter. It won't matter that is IF you have a layer of fat overlying your abs. Sure, they will get stronger, but you will never see them. Please don't hurt your back or get frustrated by doing 100 crunches a day with no success. Abdominals should be treated like any other muscle and trained with progression, focus, and intensity. They also don't need to be trained more than 2-3 times per week. I have listed my abdominal routine in the P/RR/S program at the end of this book and while not elaborate, it strengthens and tones the abs extremely well.

If you have a favorite abdominal workout keep doing it! If you shed the fat over your abs using the nutrition and cardio techniques we have outlined, you will eventually have a ripped 6-pack. Nearly all of us have a "six-pack" under our stomach fat but think sit-up after crunch will cause them to surface. If we didn't have abs, we wouldn't be able to walk, sit up, or turn around. We all have them. Still, we must train to strengthen them, like any muscle, which makes them more appealing when we do get leaner. So don't waste your time with any gimmick. Train hard, eat right, and you will find the definition you have always dreamed of.

Summary

The basics of working out for maximum fat loss include:

- Cardio 4-5 days per week in the AM or after lifting.
- Vary your cardio times but never surpass one hour.
- Alternate between HIIT and slow duration cardio-often in the same workout.
- Reduce insulin and increase GH release to maximize fat loss through diet and lifting protocols. Fat loss supplements can be a great aid when used appropriately.
- Cut Carbohydrates at night but don't forget your post workout shake of high GI carbohydrates and fast digesting protein.
- Consume BCAA and glutamine before cardio and during lifting. This will suppress cortisol and muscle breakdown.
- Abdominals should be trained like any other muscle group, but you must get leaner to see the definition in your mid section. Then and only then will you have your "six- pack."

Chapter 8

Here are the programs I have found to be most successful for gaining muscle and getting leaner. The training again is relatively simple, intense and progressive. Feel free to change body part splits and days of the week. Just remember the eight principles and how macronutrient timing and consumption are 75% of what we look like. Again, don't forget cardio, it is vital, but needs to be tailored to the goal. Want size, do less, want leanness, do more.

If on a baseline diet, I prefer to keep my nutrition consistent and increase cardio as the weeks go by to increase fat loss. Carbohydrate cycles are another option and can be used in place of a baseline diet. I have found that many prefer to start with a baseline program and move into carbohydrate cycles later. It all depends on your preferences. I think you have heard me ramble long enough. Here we go!

Nutrition Cheat Sheet:

Below are foods that I have found to be the easiest to consume and most cost effective to reach your transformation goals. While their caloric values may vary depending on your source, overall it will not make a dramatic difference in your success if you are just a little off. This way you won't be overwhelmed with counting calories, and will have a general nutrition guide at your disposal. These are the ballpark values I use to set up my nutrition programs.

Protein: *-indicates a fatty source of protein
**-protein and carbohydrate source

Food	Calories	Grams of Protein
4 oz Chicken breast	120	25
4 oz Turkey Breast	120	25
4 oz White fish or Tuna	120	25
6 Egg whites	90	25
1 Whole egg*	75	6
1 scoop Whey or Casein Protein	120-150 (varies by brand)	20-30 (varies by brand)
4 oz Salmon *	250	25
4 oz *Lean* steak *	200	25
Venison	150-200	25
½ cup Cottage Cheese **	80	13
1 cup skim milk **	80	8

Carbohydrates: complex unless noted with asterisk
*-Has some properties of simple and complex carbohydrates
**Indicates a simple carbohydrate

Food	Calories	Grams of Carbohydrates
½ cup Oatmeal (dry-before cooking)	150	30
1 slice Ezekiel bread	80	15
1 cup Brown Rice	200	40
1 piece of Fruit*	50-75	25
1 cup Green Vegetables	Doesn't count	Doesn't Count
1 tbsp Honey **	60	15
32 oz Gatorade **	200	56
2 scoops Vitargo *	250	60

Fat: some protein sources are added here, as they are also a good source of healthy fats. These are marked with an asterisk (*). *Egg yolks contain sat, poly, mono, and cholesterol*

Food (type of fat)	Calories	Grams of Fat
15 Almonds (Mono)	100	10
1 tbsp Peanut Butter(Mono)	100	10
1 tbsp Flax Seed Oil (Poly)	150	15
1 Whole Egg* (Saturated)	75	5
4 oz Salmon * (Poly)	250	15
4 oz Lean Steak * (Saturated)	200	10
15 Walnuts (Poly)	100	10

Don't Forget.........

1 hour Pre-workout: 15-20 g complex carbohydrates/40 g protein/5-10 g healthy fats

Immediately before and cont. drinking during lift: 20 g BCAA, 10 g glutamine, 10 g creatine, 20 g simple carbohydrates (I personally like 6 scoops of Scivation's Xtend in watermelon flavor with 1 tbsp Gatorade powder). If you must lose a substantial amount of body fat then you can skip the Gatorade although in most, it helps rather than hurts.

Immediately After lift: 40 g fast digesting protein and 40-60 grams of fast digesting carbohydrates; such as Gatorade, Vitargo, or even white bread.

Note: If you are trying to lose a substantial amount of body fat, you can stick to complex-low GI carbohydrates post-workout along with fast digesting protein such as whey. This will aid in fat loss by keeping insulin levels more stable. This is a _rare_ **exception though** and consuming high GI carbohydrates post-workout rarely does anything but benefit an individual after a hard workout.

Immediately before cardio: 5-10 g BCAA and 5-10 g glutamine. (I personally like 3 scoops of Scivation's Xtend in watermelon flavor)

Nutrition Program:

We need sufficient protein to repair our muscles and carbohydrates to fuel our workouts. Timing is essential. Fats are minimal as we will get the majority of our energy from carbohydrates. They are however an essential part of any successful nutrition program and should never drop below 10% of total calories. Always have a pre/post workout meal and don't forget the BCAA, glutamine and creatine as outlined during your workout. Try and limit carbohydrates late at night, drink at least a gallon of water per day, and get adequate rest. On days off from lifting you should skip the post-workout meal. This will automatically reduce the amount of calories you are consuming as it cycles carbohydrates without you even trying. If you need another meal, have 10 g of healthy fats and 20-40 g of lean protein. I take one cheat day per week, which again, alters the amount of carbohydrates I consume and prevents metabolic plateaus. Plus, it gives me something to look forward to!

Here is how I set up a basic nutrition program when getting leaner and gaining muscle is the primary goal. If size is the primary objective, I simply reduce cardio and increase the amount of carbohydrates consumed as outlined in the previous chapters. As you advance, the carbohydrate cycles outlined previously can also be used with great success. I will show you how I personally set mine up near the end of this book. Don't be afraid to give them a try.

Baseline Diet for a 200 lbs athlete:

<u>Goal:</u> *Gain Muscle/Lose Body Fat*
Total caloric goal to start with: Your BW x 13
Protein: 1.25g/lbs of body weight
Carbohydrates: 1.00 g/lbs of body weight
Fat: 0.25 g/lbs of bodyweight

<u>*Example Baseline Meal Plan for a 200 pound male athlete trying to lose body fat AND gain muscle*</u>

*(Feel free to substitute foods as you see fit)
Meal 1: 30 g complex carbohydrates/40 g protein/10-20 grams simple carbohydrates
Add 5-10 g healthy fats

½ cup oatmeal
tbsp honey or ½ cup fruit
40 g whey protein   OR   2 whole eggs with 10 egg whites (40g protein/10 g fat)
10-12 almonds

Meal 2: 30 g protein/ add 10 g healthy fats
30 g whey protein
tbsp peanut butter

Meal 3: 40 g protein/30 g complex carbohydrates/ 20 g carbohydrates from fruit
6 oz chicken
2 slices Ezekiel bread
1 piece of fruit

1 hr Pre-workout: 15-20 g complex carbohydrates/40 g protein/add 5-10 g healthy fats
1 slice Ezekiel bread
40 g whey protein
tbsp peanut butter

Start drinking pre-workout and throughout workout:
20 g BCAA
10 g glutamine
10g creatine
20 g simple carbohydrates (tbsp Gatorade powder)

Meal 4: Post Workout: 60 g "fast-digesting" carbohydrates/40 g protein
32 oz Gatorade or 2 scoops vitargo…..white bread even works!!
40 g whey

Meal 5: 40 g protein/ add 10-15 g healthy fats /green veggies (all you can eat)
8 oz salmon
Green Vegetables or salad with tbsp olive oil/vinegar

Meal 6: 30 g casein protein/add 10-15 g healthy fats
30 g casein protein powder or 1 cup low fat cottage cheese
tbsp peanut butter, flax seed oil, or 10 almonds

Approximate Totals:
Calories: 2600
260 g protein
200 g carbohydrates
50 g fat
* Eat as many green veggies as you can and desire. They will aid in stabilizing insulin levels, keep you full longer, and increase your overall health. As always, if you work hard, take one cheat meal or day per week-but be smart about it!

Program 1- P/RR/S Workout Breakdown: in parenthesis is the tempo you should use per week. The first number is the time you should take on the eccentric or negative, the next number is the amount of time at the bottom or top of a lift, the last number is how fast you should lift the weight. So for (4/0/1) you should take 4 seconds to lower the weight, no pause at the bottom, and a quick explosion to lift it back up.

Power Week: (4/0/1)

- Perform **reps in the 4-6 range**
- Focus on controlling the weight for 4 seconds on the eccentric or negative part of the lift. Doing this will not only increase the effectiveness of the lift and reduce injury, but greatly increase the time under tension.
- Immediately after reaching the bottom, begin the concentric lift. This should be performed with good form but as explosively as possible to increase motor unit firing through CNS activation.

- Rest 2-4 minutes between sets
- No advanced techniques such as partials, drop sets or super sets
- Power week will downshift the intensity, increase CNS activation, increase strength and maximize testosterone production
- Expect little "muscle pump" during the lifting session but VERY sore muscles in the days that follow.

Rep Range Week: (2/1/2)

- Perform **reps in the 7-9, 10-12, and 13-20 rep range**
- Focus on controlling the weight for 2 seconds on the eccentric *and* concentric parts of the lift. Doing this will not only increase the effectiveness of the lift and reduce injury, but greatly increase the time under tension.
- Rest 90 seconds-2 minute between sets.
- No advanced techniques such as partials, drop sets or super sets
- Rep Range week will dramatically increase the intensity, hit ALL the fast twitch fibers (type II), increase GH production, and greatly increase blood flow.
- Expect a tremendous "muscle pump" during this week.

Shock Week: (1/0/1)

- Perform **4 supersets and one drop set per body part.**
- Each rep should be smooth and controlled. The eccentric and concentric lifts should take about 1 second with no pause at the bottom (1/0/1). Find a nice, even rhythm.
- This week will test your mental fortitude and desire.

- Lactic acid, and therefore GH, will be maximally produced, which will greatly increase fat burning.
- Rest as little as possible between sets, just enough to catch your breath. No more than 1 minute!
- You will FORCE the body to change by hitting different rep ranges and using shorter rest periods.
- This is the week you should use partials, drop sets, super sets and rest pause tactics.
- I am not going to lie.......this week is tough!

After 3 weeks you will start again with Power week. Review your logbook, push more weight, and create a completely different stimulus. ***You must keep a logbook.*** Ideally, you should repeat the same workout you did three weeks previously and beat all your previous lifts. Should you find that you can't surpass your previous bests, then its time to switch exercises. After 3 full cycles I highly recommend taking a week off or lifting very lightly for one week without ever going to failure. This is to ensure that you do not become mentally fatigued and allow your joints and muscles to rest before starting again. Eric Broser's P/RR/S is a great program that I find highly effective, as well as allowing you to fully utilize all eight principles of muscle hypertrophy that we have discussed so far. You won't be disappointed!

9 WEEK P/RR/S CYCLE:

<u>Weeks 1,4,7</u>
Power Week:

CHEST/BIS/ABS-Monday

BENCH PRESS	3 X 4-6
INCLINE HAMMER PRESS	3 X 4-6
INCLINE DB FLYE	2 X 4-6
BB CURL	2 X 4-6
INCLINE CURL	2 X 4-6
CONCENTRATION CURL	2 X 4-6
CABLE CRUNCHES	3 X 4-6

QUADS/HAMS/CALVES-Tuesday

LEG PRESS or SQUATS	2 X 4-6
LUNGES	2 X 4-6
LEG EXTENSION	2 X 4-6
STIFF LEG DEADLIFT	2 X 4-6
LYING LEG CURL	2 X 4-6
LEG PRESS CALF RAISE	4 X 4-6

BACK/ABS-Thursday

PULLUPS	2 X 4-6
LAT PULLDOWNS	2 X 4-6
BENT OVER ROWS	2 X 4-6
CG SEATED CABLE OR HAMMER ROW	2 X 4-6
PULLOVERS	2 X 4-6
WEIGHTED LEG RAISES	3 X 4-6

DELTS/TRICEPS-Friday

MILITARY PRESS	3 X 4-6
LATERAL RAISES	3 X 4-6
BB UPRIGHT ROW	2 X 4-6
CG BENCH PRESS	2 X 4-6
EZ BAR EXTENSIONS (a.k.a Skull Crushers)	2 X 4-6
EZ BAR OVERHEAD EXTENSIONS (Bar or cable)	2 X 4-6

Weeks 2,5,8
Rep Range Week:

CHEST/BIS/ABS-Monday

FLAT DB BENCH PRESS	3 X 7-9
SMITH INCLINE PRESS	3 X 10-12
INCLINE DB FLYE	2 X 13-15
PECK DECK or CABLE CROSSOVERS	2 X 16-20
ALTERNATING DB CURL	2 X 7-9
INCLINE CURL	2 X 10-12
ROPE CURL	2 X 13-15
SUPPORTED STRAIGHT LEG RAISE	3 X 16-20

QUADS/HAMS/CALVES-Tuesday

DB LUNGES	2 X 7-9
SINGLE LEG LEG PRESS	2 X 10-12
LEG EXTENSION	2 X 13-15
SMITH STIFF LEG DEADLIFT	2 X 7-9
SEATED LEG CURL	2 X 10-12
LYING LEG CURL	2 X 13-15
STANDING CALF RAISE	4 X 16-20

BACK/ABS-Thursday

HAMMER OR LAT PULLDOWNS	2 X 7-9
HAMMER ROWS	2 X 7-9
T-BAR ROWS	2 X 10-12
V-HANDLE PULLDOWN	2 X 10-12
STIFF ARM PULLDOWN	2 X 13-15
WEIGHTED HYPEREXTENSION	3 X 13-15
CABLE CRUNCH (GO SIDE TO SIDE)	3 X 13-15

DELTS/TRICEPS-Friday

HAMMER OR MACHINE MILITARY PRESS	2 X 7-9
SINGLE ARM CABLE SIDE LATERAL	2 X 10-12
SHOULDER WIDTH GRIP CABLE UPRIGHT ROW	2 X 13-15 CABLE OR DB BENT LATERAL 2 X 13-15
DECLINE EZ BAR EXTENTIONS	2 X 7-9
V-BAR PUSHDOWN	2 X 10-12
OVERHEAD ONE ARM DB EXT	2 X 13-15

Weeks 3,6,9
Shock Week:

CHEST/BIS/ABS-Monday

SUPERSET: BENCH PRESS/ INCLINE DB FLYE	2 X 8-10
SUPERSET: SMITH INCLINE PRESS/ INCLINE HAMMER PRESS.	2 X 8-10
DROPSET: CABLE CROSSOVERS	1 X 10-12, DROP, 6-8 MORE
SUPERSET: BB CURL/INCLINE CURL	2 X 8-10
SUPERSET: HAMMER CURL/ROPE HAMMER CURL	2 X 8-10
DROPSET: LOW CABLE CURL	1 X 8-10, DROP, 4-6 MORE
SUPERSET: SUPPORTED KNEE-HIP RAISE/CABLE CRUNCH	2 X 12-15

QUADS/HAMS/CALVES-Tuesday

SUPERSET: LUNGES/SMITH SQUATS	2 X 8-10
SUPERSET: LEG EXTENSIONS/LEG PRESS	2 X 8-10
DROPSET: LEG EXTENSION...1 X 10-12, DROP, 6-8 MORE	
SUPERSET: LYING LEG CURL/STIFF LEG DEADLIFT	2 X 8-10
DROPSET: LYING LEG CURL	1 X 10-12, DROP, 6-8 MORE
SUPERSET: STANDING CALF/ SEATED CALF	2 X 8-10 (STANDING)/12-15 (SEATED)

BACK/ABS-Thursday

SUPERSET: LAT PULLDOWN/ PULLOVERS	2 X 8-10
SUPERSET: CG SEATED CABLE ROW/BENT OVER ROW	2 X 8-10
DROPSET: ONE ARM DB ROW	1 X 8-10, DROP, 4-6 MORE
DROPSET: HYPEREXTENSIONS	1 X 10-12 WITH WEIGHT, DROP, 6-8 MORE
SUPERSET: AB CRUNCH MACHINE/ LYING STRAIGHT LEG RAISE	2 X 12-15

DELTS/TRICEPS-Friday

SUPERSET: SMITH MILITARY PRESS/PECK DECK REV. FLY	2 X 8-10
SUPERSET: SIDE LATERAL/SEATED DB PRESS	2 X 8-10
DROPSET: SINGE ARM CABLE SIDE LATERAL	1 X 8-10, DROP, 4-6 MORE
SUPERSET: CLOSE GRIP BENCH PRESS/LYING EZ BAR EXT	2 X 8-10
SUPERSET: STANDING OVERHEAD CABLE EXT/PUSHDOWN	2 X 8-10
DROPSET: ROPE PUSHDOWN...2 X 10-12, DROP, 6-8 MORE	

Week 1-3:

Day	Lift	Cardio
Monday:	Chest/Bis/Abs	20 minutes in AM or post lifting
Tuesday:	Legs	OFF
Wednesday:	OFF	20 minutes in AM
Thursday:	Back/Abs	OFF
Friday:	Shoulders/Triceps	20 minutes in AM or post lifting
Saturday:	OFF	20 minutes in AM
Sunday:	OFF	Optional

Week 4-6:

Day	Lift	Cardio
Monday:	Chest/Bis/Abs	30 minutes in AM or post lifting
Tuesday:	Legs	OFF
Wednesday:	OFF	30 minutes in AM
Thursday:	Back/Abs	OFF
Friday:	Shoulders/Triceps	30 minutes in AM or post lifting
Saturday:	OFF	30 minutes in AM
Sunday:	OFF	Optional

Week 7-9:

Day	Lift	Cardio
Monday:	Chest/Bis/Abs	45 minutes in AM or post lifting
Tuesday:	Legs	OFF
Wednesday:	OFF	45 minutes in AM
Thursday:	Back/Abs	OFF
Friday:	Shoulders/Triceps	45 minutes in AM or post lifting
Saturday:	OFF	45 minutes in AM
Sunday:	OFF	Optional

The Carbohydrate Cycle and Other Weight Training Protocols

In addition to Eric Broser's phenomenal P/RR/S program, I wanted to include three of my favorite workouts I have used through the years. Try them out and see what you think. Remember, variability is key and don't be afraid to change things up a bit. Also, I show how I set up a carbohydrate cycle for myself, as this can be used in place of the baseline diet above. GOOD LUCK!

#1 German Volume Training:

- Select **any exercises you want but compound lifts work best.**
- Perform **10 sets of 10 reps with one exercise per body part.**
- Use **60% of your one rep max (IRM) for each exercise.**
- Rest **1-2 minutes between sets...this is a tough workout!**

Monday   (Chest/Biceps)

Tuesday   (Legs)

Thursday   (Back-Select one exercise for Lat/one for Midback)

Ex: pulldowns and rows

Friday   (Shoulders/Triceps)

Example Workout: Chest/Biceps

DB Incline Presses (max is 100 pounds x 60%=60 lbs)
1.   1x 10 with 60 lbs
2.   1x 10 with 60 lbs
3.   1x 10 with 60 lbs
4.   1x 10 with 60 lbs
5.   1x 10 with 60 lbs
6.   1x 10 with 60 lbs
7.   1x 10 with 60 lbs
8.   1x 10 with 60 lbs
9.   1x 10 with 60 lbs
10. 1x 10 with 60 lbs

Standing DB Curls (max is 60 pounds x 60%=35 lbs)
1.   1x 10 with 35 lbs
2.   1x 10 with 35 lbs
3.   1x 10 with 35 lbs
4.   1x 10 with 35 lbs
5.   1x 10 with 35 lbs
6.   1x 10 with 35 lbs
7.   1x 10 with 35 lbs
8.   1x 10 with 35 lbs
9.   1x 10 with 35 lbs
10. 1x 10 with 35 lbs

#2 Extended Tension Blast:

- Select **one exercise for mid-range, stretch, and contracted per bodypart.**
- **2 sets per exercise.**
- First **set is 8-12 reps to positive failure.**
- Rest **2 minutes and then do same weight again to failure.**
- At **failure, continue with x reps or drop sets until you can't possible do anymore.**

Monday   (Chest/Biceps)
Tuesday   (Legs)
Thursday   (Back)
Friday   (Shoulders/Triceps)

Example Workout:

Monday (Chest/Biceps):
Chest:

Press (Hammer or Bench or DB Press)	1x8-12; 1xto failure + xreps or drop
Incline or Flat Flye	1x8-12; 1xto failure + xreps or drop
Cable Cross Over	1x8-12; 1xto failure + xreps or drop

Biceps:

DB or BB Curls	1x8-12; 1xto failure + xreps or drop
Incline or Preacher curls	1x8-12; 1xto failure + xreps or drop
Concentration curls	1x8-12; 1xto failure + xreps or drop

Tuesday (Legs):
Quads/Hamstrings/Calves:

Squats/Lunges or Leg Press	1x8-12; 1xto failure + xreps or drop
Leg Extensions	1x8-12; 1xto failure + xreps or drop
Stiff Legged Deadlift	1x8-12; 1xto failure + xreps or drop
Leg Curls	1x8-12; 1xto failure + xreps or drop
Calf Raises	1x8-12; 1xto failure + xreps or drop

Thursday (Back):
Lats:

Lat Pulldowns or Pullups	1x8-12; 1xto failure + xreps or drop
Pullovers	1x8-12; 1xto failure + xreps or drop
V handle or Stiff Arm Pulldowns	1x8-12; 1xto failure + xreps or drop

Midback:

Rows (DB or BB)	1x8-12; 1xto failure + xreps or drop
Narrow Grip Cable Rows	1x8-12; 1xto failure + xreps or drop
Wide Grip Cable or T-Bar Rows	1x8-12; 1xto failure + xreps or drop

Friday (Shoulders/Triceps):
Shoulders:

DB/Smith or Military Presses	1x8-12; 1xto failure + xreps or drop
Lateral Raises or One Arm Cable Extension	1x8-12; 1xto failure + xreps or drop
Reverse Flyes	1x8-12; 1xto failure + xreps or drop

Triceps:

Close Grip Bench or Skull Crushers	1x8-12; 1xto failure + xreps or drop
Overhead Extensions (Cable/Bar or DB)	1x8-12; 1xto failure + xreps or drop
Kickbacks or Pushdowns	1x8-12; 1xto failure + xreps or drop

#3 Power/Occlusion Workout:

- Select **one exercise for mid-range, stretch, and contracted per bodypart.**
- 2 sets for midrange, 2 for stretch and 1 set for contracted.
- Midrange **sets are 2x 4-6 reps to positive failure.**
- Stretch **are 2 x 10-12 reps to positive failure plus x reps or drop after 2**nd **set.**
- Contracted **is one set of 20-40 reps to failure!!!!!!**
- Rest **2 minutes after each set.**

Monday   (Chest/Biceps)

Tuesday   (Legs)

Thursday   (Back)

Friday   (Shoulders/Triceps)

Example Workout:

Monday (Chest/Biceps):

Chest:

Press (Hammer or Bench or DB Press)	2x4-6 to failure
Incline or Flat Flye	1x8-12; 1xt8-12 to failure + xreps
Cable Cross-Over	1x20-40 to failure

Biceps:

DB or BB Curls	2x4-6 to failure
Incline or Preacher curls	1x8-12; 1x8-12 failure + xreps
Concentration curls	1x20-40 to failure

Tuesday (Legs):

Quads/Hamstrings/Calves:

Squats/Lunges or Leg Press	2x4-6 to failure
Stiff Legged Deadlift	1x8-12; 1x8-12 failure + xreps
Leg Extensions	1x20-40 to failure
Leg Curls	1x8-12; 1xto failure + xreps or drop
Calf Raises	1x8-12; 1xto failure + xreps or drop

Thursday (Back):

Lats:

Lat Pulldowns or Pullups	2x4-6 to failure
Pullovers	1x8-12; 1x8-12 failure + xreps
V handle or Stiff Arm Pulldowns	1x20-40 to failure

Midback:

Rows (DB or BB)	2x4-6 to failure
Narrow Grip Cable Rows	1x8-12; 1x8-12 failure + xreps
Wide Grip Cable or T-Bar Rows	1x20-40 to failure

Friday (Shoulders/Triceps):

Shoulders:

DB/Smith or Military Presses	2x4-6 to failure
Lateral Raises or One Arm Cable Extension	1x8-12; 1x8-12 failure + xreps
Bent Over Reverse Flyes	1x20-40 to failure

Triceps:

Close Grip Bench or Skull Crushers	2x4-6 to failure
Overhead Extensions (Cable/Bar or DB)	1x8-12; 1x8-12 failure + xreps
Kickbacks or Pushdowns	1x20-40 to failure

Carbohydrate Cycle

Here is how I set up a carbohydrate cycle. This is a breakdown of cycle 1, but cycle 2 is also very productive. Feel free to use various foods, as these are the ones that I prefer. Nobody should be miserable-so find the set-up that works best for you.

Monday: Medium

Tuesday: High

Wednesday: Low

Thursday: Medium

Friday: Medium

Saturday: Low

Sunday: High (cheat day)

Low Carbohydrate Days: 2 days

Bodyweight (200) x 0.5=100 g carbohydrate for the day
Bodyweight(200) x 1.5= 300 g protein for the day
Bodyweight (200) x 0.35 = 70 g fat for the day

- No fruit allowed
- Spread these out over 6-8 meals and try to get most of your carbohydrates before 3 PM

Meal 1: 50 g complex carbohydrates/50 g lean protein

1 cup oatmeal
Splenda for flavor
2 scoops whey protein

Meal 2: 50 g lean protein/ add 15 g healthy fats/ vegetables
8-10 oz chicken/tuna or turkey
Handful almonds
Veggies

Meal 3: 50 g complex carbohydrates/50 g lean protein/veggies
8-10 oz chicken or turkey
1 cup brown rice
Veggies

Meal 4: 50 g lean protein/ add 15 g healthy fats
2 scoops whey
1 tbsp PB

Meal 5: 50 g protein/ add 15 g healthy fats/green vegetables
8-10 oz meat (if steak or salmon, then hold off on olive oil)
Salad with olive oil/vinegar as dressing

Meal 6: 50 g casein/whey protein/ add 15 g healthy fats
1 scoop whey/ 1scoop casein or mixed protein blend with tbsp peanut butter

Medium Carbohydrate Days: 3 days
Bodyweight (200) x 1= 200 carbohydrate in grams for the day
Bodyweight(200) x 1.5= 300 protein in grams fir the day
Bodyweight (200) x .25 = 50 fat in grams for the day

- One piece of fruit allowed at meal 1 and 2
- Spread these out over 6-8 meals and try to get most of your carbohydrates before 7 PM

Meal 1: 30 g complex carbohydrates/15 g simple carbs/50 g lean protein

1/2 cup oatmeal
Tbsp honey
2 scoop whey

Meal 2: 50g lean protein/25 g carbohydrates from fruit or milk
1 cup cottage cheese/ 1 scoop whey with 1-2 cup fruit

Meal 3: 50 g lean protein/40 g complex carbohydrates/veggies
8-10 oz lean meat
1 cup brown rice
Veggies

1 hr Pre-workout: 15 g complex carbohydrates/10 g xtra fat/25 g whey
protein
1 slices Ezekial bread w/tbsp natural PB/ 1 scoop whey

15 minutes pre-workout and throughout workout:
20 g BCAA
10 g glutamine
10g creatine
20 g simple carbohydrates (Tbsp Gatorade powder)

Meal 4: Post Workout: 60 g "fast" carbohydrates/40 g whey protein
32 oz Gatorade or 2 scoops vitargo
40 g whey

Meal 5: 25 g "fatty" protein/green vegetables
4 oz salmon or steak
Add veggies

Meal 6: 25 g casein protein/ add 15 g healthy fats
1 scoop casein or mixed protein blend with tbsp peanut butter

High Carbohydrate Days: 2 days- <u>if you have a cheat day it counts as a
high day</u>

Bodyweight (200) x 1.5-1.75=300 carbohydrate in grams for the day
Bodyweight(200) x 1= 200 protein in grams for the day
Bodyweight (200) x .25 = 50 fat in grams for the day

- one piece of fruit allowed with each meal but NEVER after working out.
- Schedule at least one high day per week on leg day…you'll need it!
- Spread these out over 6-8 meals and try to get most of your carbohydrates before 7 PM

Meal 1: 50-60 g complex carbohydrates/15 g simple carbs/25 g lean protein

1 cup oatmeal
Tbsp honey
1 scoop whey

Meal 2: 25g lean protein/25 g carbohydrates from fruit or milk
1 cup cottage cheese with 2 cup fruit

Meal 3: 25 g lean protein/50 g complex carbohydrates/veggies
4 oz lean meat
1 cup brown rice
Veggies

1 hr Pre-workout: 30 g complex carbohydrates/10 g xtra fat/25 g whey protein
½ cup oatmeal or 2 slices Ezekial bread w/tbsp natural PB
1 scoop whey protein

15 minutes pre-workout and throughout workout:
20 g BCAA
10 g glutamine
10g creatine
20 g simple carbohydrates (Tbsp Gatorade powder)

Meal 4: Post Workout: 60 g "fast" carbohydrates/40 g whey protein
32 oz Gatorade or 2 scoops vitargo
40 g whey

Meal 5: 25 g lean protein/40 g complex carbohydrates/green vegetables
4 oz meat
1 cup whole wheat pasta or brown rice
Add veggies

Meal 6: 25 g casein protein/ add 15 g healthy fats
1 scoop casein or mixed protein blend with tbsp peanut butter

By now, you should understand how to manipulate your training, caloric intake, and macronutrients to meet your goals. These are the basic workouts and nutrition programs I use most often. If an individual wants to get bigger, they should increase calories and decrease cardio accordingly. The opposite of course is true if one wishes to get leaner. No matter the goal, I believe you should still take a cheat day but decrease them as your deadline approaches.

The workout mentality stays the same. Lift hard and intensely no matter the goal. Record everything. That way you will know where to make changes. You already know the how. Please know that you can structure these workouts to suit you as an individual. If you hate bench presses, do dumbbell presses, if you have back problems, don't do heavy squats. There are always ways to work around injuries and keep making gains. Practice the eight principles and incorporate them into P/RR/S or the workouts of your choice. Substituting into these workouts is easy and I actually advise you all to change lifts frequently, no matter the program. Below, I have included three questions you should ask yourself at the end of every day while on your quest to transform your body. They have helped me more than you can imagine.

What was one thing I did very well today?

What was one thing I could have done better today?

What is one thing I'll do better tomorrow?

Conclusions

First, I want to thank all of you for taking the time to read this book. It was a goal of mine to help those who desired to make a change. Please realize it is more a possibility than a dream. I hope it gives you a solid start towards transforming your body and reaching your goals. Never stop asking questions and never give up on what you as an individual truly want to accomplish. I promise you can get there. Stay in touch and let me know if you have any questions or thoughts. I can be reached at eyady@hotmail.com. Train hard and make the most of each day your given.

All the Best,

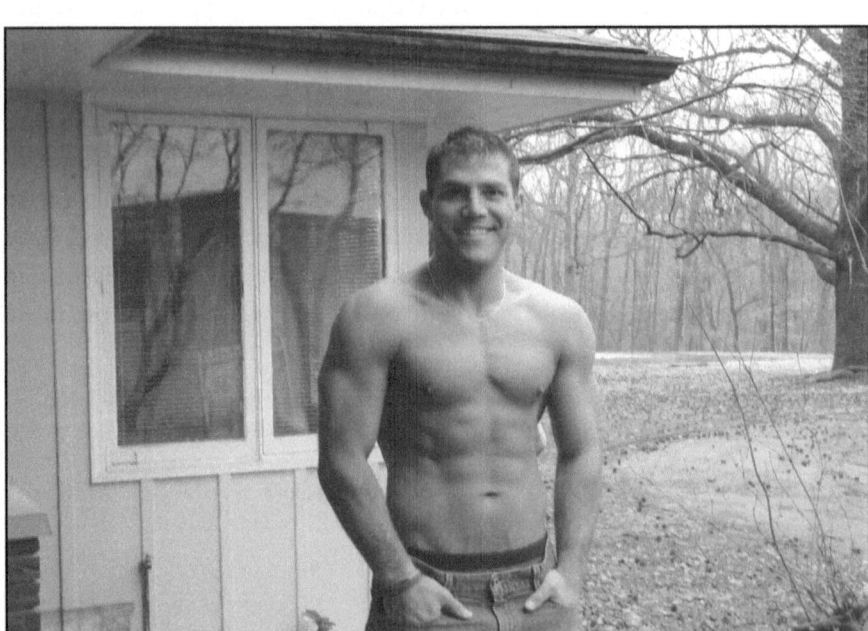

www.ingramcontent.com/pod-product-compliance
Lightning Source LLC
Chambersburg PA
CBHW020912290526

45784CB00002BA/518